The Book of Walking

An exploration of the many adventures of a walk

by
Robert L. Cain

Property News Service

Oro Valley, Arizona

The Book of Walking

Copyright 2020

By Robert L. Cain

Cover Design and photo by Robert L. Cain

Dedication

To wife Marilyn, my children Cody and Laurel, and my grandchildren Victoria and Brendan with whom my walks have always been a joy.

Contents

Introduction

It started out as Zen Walking. That was the title I chose and aimed at as the chapters progressed. But things got in the way such as the history of walking, competitive walking, and guilt walking. Still others had to be pounded into a hole too small to fit the scope of the chapter. After all, seeing-if-you-can walking can include being mindful, and in fact, I discuss that in Chapter 6, but it better fits as physical accomplishment. I had to figure out a way for the scope of the book to encompass all the combinations and permutations of a walk. After all, that cogitation and rumination I had to change the title and the subtitle while still doing justice to the Zen part because freeing your mind, resetting your brain, turning off anxiety, and seeing the world differently are still wonderful reasons to set foot out the door.

One day I came up with a subtitle that fit the bill. I wrote about it in the Ruminating Walking chapter. Was that a Zen experience? I suppose it depends on how you define Zen experience. That's another idea I thought about discussing: how do you define Zen? Are there rules we must follow? I say no, but I'm not big on rules and regulations. It's just whatever works. Instead, I needed a different word to describe what one's mind does on a walk, or what one wants one's mind to do. After writing down 40 or so possible words and sitting with the thesaurus for a couple of hours, I came up with a word I believe encompasses what I have aimed at with Zen, reflective. Mostly rumination, seeing and observing, mindfulness, and joyful walking have to do with reflection. But that still didn't work, so back to the lists of words and examinations of the thesaurus.

After two weeks of finding words that wouldn't work, including reflective, I arrived at the word that best encompasses the goal and results of what walking does for the mind. I had passed over this word without thinking about it despite the fact that it appeared in just about every search I did for words that would work. The Oxford English Dictionary defines it as "Power or exercise of vision; look, gaze," and "Mental perception or recognition." The word is ken. That's a word unfamiliar to most people unless you watch "Outlander." But the Scots use it as a verb meaning to know. Ken, in this case, is a noun, where you have vision and mental perception.

Ken encompasses the philosophy I expound in the book as far as a walk being mind-expanding and mind-freeing. No matter, though, a good walk is an individual, a personal experience. I have no business telling anyone how fast, how far, when how, or where anyone should walk or what you should get from a walk. I can only describe what works for me—most of the time, anyway. That isn't necessarily what will work for anyone else. If it does, great. If it doesn't, try something else until you hit on your formula for a good walk. That may change as walks accumulate and you find something you like better. Nothing is or needs to be forever or made into an arbitrary rule. There are those, "experts," who prescribe what you should do on a walk and the reasons for going for a walk. I just don't agree. The careful research I have conducted for this book shows that even the experts and the studies are often at odds. Hence, here's only what works for me.

All that said, in this book you will find 12 ½ reasons to go for a walk. If any of these work for you, that pleases me. No matter if you just decide to go for one walk because of what you read here; that pleases me, too.

The 12 Principles

1. Every walk is a new adventure

2. Enjoy and relish each moment of a walk.

3. Counting steps can be a trap. There's no "magic" number of steps for health. In fact, the mantra advice they give has no basis in the science of physiology. Plus, it can trample the enjoyment of the world and the walk and push you to overdo.

4. It takes a while to learn your limitations, so pay attention to what your body says. It's easy to overdo, so walk less than you might be tempted.

5. Walking in nature is especially rewarding because it resets the brain, there's no traffic or crowds, and the air is fresher.

6. Sometimes a walk isn't fun or enjoyable, or particularly rewarding, but it's better than sitting at a desk in front of a computer screen or on the couch in front of a TV.

7. Guilt is a falsehearted, perfidious motivator.

8. Guilt can rear its ugly head if you walk only for exercise.

9. Curiosity could conceivably get you in trouble, but the satisfaction of what you discover makes it memorable.

10. Watch your step. An injury can ruin a perfectly good day, week, or month.

11. It's nothing to brag about, only to relish. There's no contest here. You don't have to "get there," be faster, or walk longer unless you want to. The walk is its own reward.

12. Great minds think a hike. (This one I saw on a bumper sticker and couldn't resist.)

Chapter 1

The Adventure Awaits

After a frantic search, my mother found me, 18 months old, walking down the middle of a state highway. It was my first grand adventure. It's about a half mile from where we lived in Portland to US 26, Powell Blvd., and I walked it—all alone. I have no recollection of it whatsoever, but my mother occasionally reminded me, so I will have to take her word for it. It must have been my initiation into rambling, for seeing the world, for satisfying my almost insatiable curiosity, for my thirst for seeing what's around the next corner, of what's on the next block, of what's down that path. This one was just a herald of hundreds of adventures to come, some more grand than others, and a sign of my penchant for exploration.

The map shows I had to turn two corners and cross at least one street to get to Powell. No parent or grandparent was there to interfere with my adventure. Just exploring. I am certain some brand new and fascinating sights soaked into my brain. They're lost now. I just went to see what I could see.

It wasn't as bad as it sounds. Even though Powell was a highway, the kind with a line down the middle of it and a posted speed limit, and signs indicating it was US 26, it does not begin to compare with the four-lane, center turn-lane state highway it is now. In old photos, it almost looks like a side street. In fact, I believe I have lived on streets busier than Powell Blvd. was at that time, such as Grant St. in Denver where my wife and I lived years later. But there I was, checking out the line in the middle of Powell Blvd. Where had my mother been? How did I get so far away before she found me? I never heard that part of the story.

That first grand exploratory adventure was just the beginning with hundreds more to come. Some of my most memorable walks I'll talk about in a minute. Walking has been my passion ever since I took my first steps at 13 months old. With the power to get places on my own and independent cuss that I am, I didn't need to depend on a parent to push me in a stroller, carry me, or hold my hand. After those beginnings of freedom, I sometimes was more free than others might have preferred.

Much of the attraction of walking for me is that I experience the world. Stopping to look at some newly discovered attraction or changed attraction, to wander off the path to satisfy my curiosity about some new sight or route or even to explore farther are all possibilities I delight in. Think how much we miss when the world whizzes by at the speed of running or bicycling. But if someone walks solely for exercise and won't stop lest the exercise be ruined, it may work for that person but I think misses the best parts of a walk. Walking for exercise, as we'll look at in Chapter 15, eventually ends up with a discouraged walker.

I have ridden a bicycle 100 miles at a time; I have run four marathons and done all the daily training required to run the 26.2 miles. In addition, I have run numerous 10Ks and 5Ks. Of course, I had to train just about daily to run any of those. But in all that training, rarely, if ever, did I stop to see stuff, It's far more so in the case of running than with bicycling because we run for a different reason than experiencing the world. It is for exercise or maybe for an experience (that almost never happens) where you float above the pavement.

> *But the walking of which I speak has nothing in it akin to taking exercise, as it is called, as the sick take medicine at stated hours—as the swinging of dumbbells or chairs; but is itself the enterprise and adventure of the day.—Henry David Thoreau,* "Walking"

Just about every day I have an adventure now, maybe grand, maybe not. The potential for adventure is infinite, even just across the parking lot from the car to the store. It can be the highlight of the day, the activity I wake up in the morning thinking about, the plan I make for my daily adventure. Sometimes I wake up thinking about where I am going to walk that day, what new sights and sites I may see.

During the summer heat, I hop, step tentatively, or creak out of bed early ready to be astonished by the adventure. Other days I wonder if I am sure I want to walk or would just rather make my way downstairs, eat breakfast, and drink coffee. But I am nearly always pleased when I do walk, or at least pat myself on the back that I did.

Let's go for a walk. No, let's go for lots of walks. I have come up with 13 ways to go for a walk, and some of them easily combine to do double or even triple duty. I'll look at each of these ways in the following pages and tell stories about them along with some interesting side trips—that may be more interesting than the walks themselves. We'll see. I am certain at least one these ways will work for you to make an anticipate walk an adventure as they work for me.

Contemplative walking.

I almost always walk alone but not mournfully as in the song by Sammy Cahn "I'll Walk Alone. "They'll ask me why and I'll tell them I'd rather. There are dreams I must gather." Yes, I'd rather. Many people prefer to walk with a partner or a group, and it works for them, but I usually don't want to walk with anyone but family and close friends, or with someone else when we have something to discuss that is better done on foot.

For me "there are dreams [and thoughts] I must gather." The main reason I walk alone is that I work when I walk. In the past, it may have been a time for me to explore without interruption or having to deal with what someone else wanted to see, or just to be alone with my thoughts, impressions, and explorations (explorations being one of my favorite walking pretexts and one that often extends a walk). Some impressions and thoughts have stuck with me and only get rummaged up out of memory when a recollection jumps out and latches on to my consciousness. I never know what will stick with me forever including the stories my brain manufactures about the things I see.

Seeing and Observing

One extraordinary thing I discovered is that walking has made me better at "seeing." Before I started thinking about becoming better at "seeing" and more observant, I didn't notice some of the things I do now. Awareness of the world is one treasured perk of a walk, one that rewards with memories that repay the effort maybe even decades after. It echoes Thoreau's observation he wrote in "Walking," "Some of my townsmen, it is true, can remember and have described to me some walks which they took ten years ago, in which they were so blessed as to lose themselves for half an hour in the woods." Too bad he adds a zinger berating them for sticking to walking on roads ever since. Walking in nature has several benefits as shown in a study we'll look at in Chapter 5 on "Ruminating Walking." But not now.

I have countless memories about walking both in nature and on city streets that have lasted decades. This is what walking does for me. If it can do something for you, terrific. Everyone walks for his or her own reasons and at (and because of) his or her own comfort level. And those reasons are that person's, no one else's. They are neither right nor wrong but simply are. They are each individual's reasons, and they are not mine to judge, well, at least out loud. If what you read here inspires a walk, that pleases me. If you just enjoy reading the book, that pleases me, too. In fact, if you buy the book that pleases me just as much and maybe even more.

Exploratory Walking

I was by no means finished exploring and ruminating after my first grand adventure at 18 months old. My first actual recollection of wanderlust adventuring occurred when I was four years old. My parents had moved to Burns, Oregon, in a house across the street from open fields with sage brush, coyotes, and rattlesnakes. I must have been bored what with all the moving in activity, and curious, as is my wont, because I started off into the field on my exploration. I remember it was daylight when I started, but then it was dark. I turned around in the direction I had come but couldn't see my new house, or any house for that matter with my four-year-old's view blocked by head-high sage brush, as though I could have remembered what it looked like after just a few hours there. My four-year-old brain got confused.

With the way to my new home not obvious, I remember wandering around until I saw a house with lights on. Not the least bit shy, I knocked on the door and told them that I was lost, my name, and that my father worked at Penney's. They got in touch with my parents who came and got me. I suppose they were relieved I didn't get bitten by a rattle snake or eaten by a hungry coyote.

A couple of years later, we moved to Chula Vista, California, and in grade school I walked about a mile alone to school every day. We lived a block too close to the one mile limit for the school bus to pick me up, but that was a matter of complete indifference to me since I had never ridden a school bus. I suppose now, there's no way a six-year-old would be allowed to walk to school alone. A parent would have driven me to school, but my mother didn't drive and my father was at work. Oh, well, what a lucky stroke and what fascinating experiences that introduced the world to me. One etched memory occurred as I was walking home one day past a truck farm. I suppose with my innate curiosity I had stood and watched the men work for a while. One of the men called me over and offered me a stalk of freshly picked celery. That may be the best celery I have ever eaten. I keep waiting for celery to taste that good again.

After our move back to Portland, I walked to my grandparents' house, often alone, but sometimes with my brother. I didn't know how far it was until I looked it up on a measure distance on a map website. It is a little over a mile with several route options providing many exploratory opportunities.

I have an almost unerring sense of direction, despite my having gotten turned around when I was four years old, but that was not the case with my younger brother. One of the instructions to him was "turn right at the red door." I don't know if I ever was conscious of a red door, or even thought about it again until I wrote this. No red door required for me to get to my grandparents' house and back again.

High school required a city bus to get to school. Most days I took the bus both ways, an experience that is lost in the blur of memory—always the same and always unmemorable except for the amusing time the police stopped the bus and gave the driver a ticket for some infraction or other. But those days when I walked home, I was able to keep in touch with the city. It was about three-and-a-half miles with a myriad of available routes. A friend lived about a mile from school and I sometimes walked part way with him then went on my own the rest of the way. Had I known what I know now, I would have made notes as I walked, but a 16-year-old brain, even a 16-year-old writer's brain, didn't make the connection with keeping notes to remember what I saw and experienced. Live and learn.

Rumination Walking

The best part of where I lived in high school, though, was Mt. Tabor, the 195-acre city park three houses away from my front door. Spending countless hours exploring the hills in the park, and they were and are considerable, I am sure I discovered every inch of the park, all the side paths and main paths, all the roads and trails, all the off-trail nooks and crannies. I got to walk alone and it delivered me chances to be left alone to ruminate on whatever I wanted to ruminate on, what with parents who were none too kind and two brothers and a sister at home. Rumination is something we will look at extensively in another chapter.

> *A lone walker is both present and detached from the world around, more than an audience but less than a participant. Walking assuages or legitimizes this alienation: one is mildly disconnected because one is walking, not because one is incapable of connecting." –* *Rebecca Solnit,* Wanderlust

In college, after escaping the dorm, far more prodigious walks awaited me, including one that tripled after I moved even farther from the college. Every day I walked through Lithia Park in Ashland, Oregon, on the way to and from school or into downtown. It didn't get much better than that. My wife and I recently visited Ashland as part of an anniversary trip and walked through Lithia Park, just as we had daily years earlier. And it had changed. I marveled at how the city of Ashland had made the path steeper than it had been decades before. They had to move all that dirt, those mature trees, and large structures to increase the grade. Even so, it was a wonderful walk, one we did twice, and it brought back many of the feelings and memories we had had when it was our daily walk.

Social Walking

As an adult what I remember as to size and distance is mostly accurate, though the farther back in time it is, the less accurate it becomes. Even so, some walks seemed like no distance at all. Some of my fondest memories are of the walks we took in Forest Park. Portland's Forest Park with over 5,000 acres is one of the largest urban forests in the United States. It has more than 80 miles of unpaved trails, fire lanes and forest roads. For seven miles it overlooks Northwest Portland, and in some places overlooks the Willamette River. The northern end provides a view of where the Columbia and Willamette Rivers come together on the way to the Pacific Ocean.

When my children were growing up, we regularly enjoyed Forest Park. They could run and explore to their hearts' content, savoring the wilderness only a half hour by car from home. One of the best parts of those walks was our dog Oliver. Our children ran ahead on the trail, with Oliver hot on their heels. After a while, he would come running back to my wife and me to make sure we were still coming, then run back to the kids again. We went probably once a month, always looking forward to it. I didn't walk alone there, but walking with others in Forest Park was truly rewarding.

Distances vary from a mile or so to 12 miles on Leif Erickson Dr. We had our favorites, but over time the specific routes have become lost to memory. I always remember, though, the smell of the Douglas Fir and the solid clumps of bracken fern that line the trails. It's a place you want to return to over and over. You see something new every visit, even on the same trails.

After my children were grown and gone, my wife and I decided that we would walk every Forest Park trail on weekends. We got many of them re-explored before the fall rains set in.

Now, from just outside of Tucson, I walk every day and every walk is a new adventure whether it's as I work or even to a store anywhere from 20 to 45 minutes.

There's something about walking that connects with the world that driving, riding a bike, or even running can't. Feet touch earth or pavement and move at a pace just right for seeing the world. You can stop and look, observe, enjoy, see, and contemplate what you experience without the guilt of interrupting your "exercise" or need to "get there." However, it seems if I have   specific destination, I walk faster than I would prefer. When I walk just for walking's sake, I don't need to "get there," only to "be there," wherever "there" is.

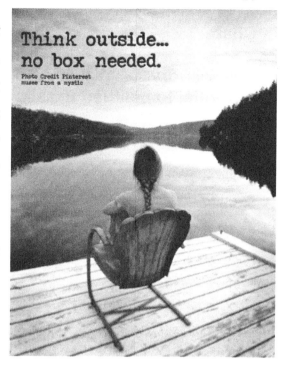

**Think outside...
no box needed.**

Photo Credit Pinterest
musee from a mystic

That's what this book is about, the experience of walking in all its permutations and combinations so we can experience the world at our own pace and for our own reasons.

Itching for another adventure, I feel a walk coming on.

Chapter 2

The History of Walking, or how it went from essential to belittled to respected

Until turnpikes, it was okay to walk to get from one place to another. Even then, though, pedestrians' acceptability was fading fast. For eons, walking was the only or by far most common way to get from one place to another, but over time, its purpose and repute evolved (or devolved). Here's how its respectability was lost to modern progress.

They began in 1663 and built up steam until they peaked in England as "turnpike mania" from 1750 to 1772. Turnpikes were privately built and funded toll roads. Such a potentially profitable idea awaiting and not wanting to miss out, Americans began to build turnpikes with the first ones completed in 1792. They multiplied rapidly both in England and America as people appreciated a more reliable way to drive their carts and carriages. Of course there were tolls to pay for them and they varied as to the location and the type of vehicle, but pedestrians walked free, and that apparently was the rub.

Turnpikes' history is interesting both in the US and England, but they were created because getting around on the rutted, uneven, muddy roads was just too much of an imposition for those who came to expect they should get more easily from one place to another in wheeled vehicles. Trade and travel is much more efficient in vehicles that roll on wheels. Investors, write Donald Klein and John Majewski in their paper "Turnpikes and Toll Roads in Nineteenth Century America," didn't get or expect much of a monetary return, but rather "returns in use and esteem rather than cash." In fact, Frederick Wood wrote in his 1919 book *Turnpikes of New England*, "it seems to have been generally known long before the rush of construction subsided that turnpike stock was worthless." But they were a boon "to merchants, farmers, land owners, and ordinary residents," wrote Klein and Majewski because they offered "indirect benefits" because "everyone feels that he has been repaid for his expenditures in the improved value of his lands, and the economy of business."

The major advantage was not just the roads themselves; roads existed before, but now the roads were maintained so that wheeled vehicles and horses could reliably traverse them without so much concern about getting stuck in ruts and the mud or overturning because of such things as tree roots. In Chapter 12 we'll take a look at how the aristocracy dealt with the problem of bad roads with their footmen running and walking alongside the carriages and how footmen became the source of a new gambling game.

What all that means is that the toll roads were there to benefit those who could afford to pay, the middle class and wealthy. After all, they invested in and built the turnpikes.

Where did that leave the walkers? They didn't have to pay, after all. People in England increasingly began to look askance on those who walked, albeit with a smidgen of justification, but one expanded to make all walkers suspect, because criminals could also more easily escape on foot in densely populated urban and forested areas.

Once horse travel and especially carriage travel became *de rigueur*, it was positively silly to travel any distance on foot. After all, only those who didn't have the money to buy or rent even a horse walked where they were going except for those who had reasons to walk that didn't necessarily include travel (more about that in a moment).

The English came up with a name for these walkers, "pikeys." The word has a dual origin, one that refers to the walking stick used by turnpike walkers. In this case, the word "pike" is a verb, figuratively "to pike oneself meant to travel on foot, go away, or run away," explains Douglas Wilson on worldwidewords.org. The other origin is "pikers," the shortened version of "turnpikers."

The word pikey is still a slang term in England referring to "travelers," those people with no permanent place of abode—and also the Irish. A derivative is also a slang term in the US, "piker," meaning "a vagrant, tramp, or good-for-nothing." There is some debate about its origin in this country.

One theory for the American term is the same one as the one in England, where walkers, who walked free on turnpikes, were called turnpikers, later shortened to "pikers." They were denigrated because, after all, anyone who had to walk rather than ride must be suspect.

A second American theory of the word's origin comes from the former residents of Pike County, Missouri, who took off on foot heading for the gold fields of California in 1849. They were apparently a rag-tag bunch much as Okies were during the Depression bailing out of the Midwest and the dustbowl.

A small minority walked because for a variety of reasons they wanted to. In the years just before 1800, walking any distance had become so belittled that William Wordsworth and his sister Dorothy were looked down upon for mostly walking from Stockton, England, to their new home Dove Cottage near Grasmere in the Lake District, a distance of almost 100 miles. It took them four days and included side trips to see waterfalls and other sights. Dorothy Wordsworth wrote *The Grasmere Journals* that someone who traveled for pleasure absent a hired coach or on horseback was assumed to be either lacking the money for a coach or horse or basic sanity. The Wordsworths did travel part of the way on horseback, though, thus restoring some of their perceived sanity, I suppose.

Dorothy Wordsworth, in a letter to her aunt in 1794, wrote, "I cannot pass unnoticed that part of your letter in which you speak of my 'rambling about the country on foot.' So far from considering this as a matter of condemnation, I rather thought it would have given my friends pleasure to hear that I had courage to make use of the strength with which nature has endowed me, when it not only procured me infinitely more pleasure than I should have received from sitting in a post chaise— but was also the means of saving me at least thirty shillings." That's about 155 pounds in today's English currency.

Karl Philip Moritz (1756-1793), a German minister, spent seven weeks in 1782 traveling across England, bringing with him his book of Milton's *Paradise Lost*. He wanted to experience Milton where Milton began. That was Milton in one pocket and clean linen in the other, no other baggage. He traveled light. Three of the weeks he was in London. There he attracted no derision, but in the hinterland, he "often found himself scorned and ejected by innkeepers and their employees, while coachmen and carters continually asked him if he wanted a ride," writes Rebecca Solnit in her book *Wanderlust*. Moritz wrote, "a traveler on foot in this country seems to be considered as a sort of wild man, or an out-of-the-way-being, who is stared at, pitied, suspected, and shunned by everybody who meets him." You see, as he reported in his travel essays, "everybody who was anybody rode."

Riding was not always the best option for him, though. It turns out that walking was safer. On one coach he rode on the roof and feared for his life as the coach careened down a hill. He did discover that how he was treated in inns sometimes depended on if he drank with the landlord and toasted his health. At one inn, everyone had toasted to his health and apparently everyone else's, but Moritz missed the clue and didn't toast to anyone's health, not even the landlord's. His stay at that inn was less than pleasant. From that day forward, in every inn, he drank to "Your healths, gentlemen all."

His less-than-welcoming greetings might also have had to do with his appearance, traveling light as he was. In London, it was not so much an issue, but after a couple of weeks of wearing the same clothes, he had to look just a little unkempt. That might be especially the case after the hill climb he described in one essay where he slipped in the mud. Showing up at an inn in that condition could well have been off-putting to local residents. The English weren't big on baths in those days, but they did wear relatively clean clothes.

To his credit, the young man kept his faith in the English character and reported his ill-usage in his essays with no bitterness.

He did well in life as friend of Johann von Goethe, Friederich Schiller, and Johann Georg Herder, and as professor of archaeology and aesthetics at the Berlin Academy of Art, and as a member of the Prussian Academy of Sciences. He wrote *Essay toward a Practical Logic for Children* in 1786 and edited the *Magazine for Empirical Psychology.* All this from a man who spent seven weeks tromping around England with only Milton's *Paradise Lost* in one pocket and linen in the other, experiencing what it was like to travel on foot in England.

The denigration of walking gets even worse. I found "25 Words for Walking" with 17 of them that could be considered derogatory, some not even "could be" but are derogatory. Careen, falter, flounder, lumber, lurch, meander, prowl, ramble, saunter, skulk, stagger, stumble, totter, parade, and waddle all have derogatory connotations. So many words to describe walking pejoratively. Drivers are off the hook, though. In an article on oppositelock.kinja.com, "We need a catch-all term, a common slur for bad drivers. We call motorcycle riders with no gear *Squids,* and it is pretty universally understood." I must not be part of the universe because I had never heard or seen the word "squids" to describe anything but sea creatures. The article could not come up with any particular common derogatory term for a motorist, though. Maybe you can think of a few, but none appeared in the article. So pedestrians can have aspersions cast upon them in at least 17 ways, but motorists get off scot free.

Lest you think that words such as meander, prowl, saunter, stumble, totter and waddle preceded their use as derogatory terms for walking, the word "meander, for example, came to be used as a derogatory term in 1746 to mean what it does now, "to wander about aimlessly." It also is of common derivation to "maunder," which comes from "maund," which means to beg.

Even "parade," as innocent as that might seem at first glance, has one meaning from 1656 "to show ostentation or bravado." Saunter is another that took on a derogatory meaning about 1725, meaning "lounge; idle occupation," reports the Oxford English Dictionary (OED).

Then there is the word "pedestrian." According to Isabel Colgate in her book *A Pelican in the Wilderness*, the word was not used before it referred to Wordsworthian travels. Before that, if someone roamed the countryside, "he was referred to as a hermit, a shepherd, a tradesman, or an inhabitant of a post-chaise," writes Trina-Marie Baird in her paper on Wordsworth's walking.

However, the word "pedestrianism" had an entirely respectable meaning. Those hardy souls engaged in the sport of "pedestrianism" were heroes beginning in England in the late 18th and early 19th Centuries and later in the US, earning considerable money and respect for their efforts. I will describe them and their feats in Chapter 12 about competitive walking.

Of particular interest is the word "transient." The OED shows its first usage in 1607, but meaning "Passing by or away with time; not durable or permanent; temporary, transitory; esp. passing away quickly or soon, brief, momentary, fleeting." It took a couple of hundred years until the late 19th Century for it to acquire its present colloquial usage as "A person who passes through a place, or stays in it only for a short time; . . . a traveler, a tramp, a migrant worker." When we speak of people today as transients, we speak of them in a less-than-favorable light. The word still holds its original adjectival meaning, but as a noun, it says bum.

It was at about this time, the turn of the 19th Century, that walking for pleasure was becoming acceptable, though not for travel as English usage indicates. Even today, the English language consigned walking and pedestrians to something less than desirable. For example, traffic engineers have given them the designations of "pedestrian impedance," or "vehicular delay."

Of course, for millennia, walking for travel was the only way to get around. It wasn't until between 4500 and 2000 BC (no one knows for sure) that horses, the first method of non-walking transportation, were even domesticated. And even then, they weren't for riding when they were first penned up and tamed in what is now the steppes of Southern Russia and the Ukraine.

For thousands of years before, horses were hunted for food. Even after domestication, they were still sometimes food; it was just easier to get dinner from a pen than from hunting. Even at that, mankind had to wait until farming became prevalent because hunter gatherers simply had no place to keep horses. But horses were smaller 6,000 years ago and had to be bred to get them large enough to ride. Until then, they were used as animals that could carry stuff in far greater quantities than people could.

Walking was still the default method of travel even after horses were made part of domestic society because obviously domestication took a while to spread into Europe and Asia and never did get to North America until the Spanish, Portuguese and English explorers brought horses.

But horse travel was the beginning of the end for walking as the default means of travel, at least for the more affluent. I mean, why not? People can travel much farther, much faster on a horse than on foot, and they can run down game far more efficiently, and of course, have an overwhelming advantage in battle against a foe who is on foot.

Other animals had been domesticated before the horse, cows, goats, sheep, but none of them lends itself to load bearing. Oxen were perhaps the exception because they could pull things such as wagons and plows, but they are neither for riding nor for carrying things. Cows, goats, and sheep provide milk, wool, and food. Horses are almost designed to work as transportation and pack animals because of the interdental space that provides a perfect slot for a bit, making them easier to control.

But back to walking gaining acceptability. The idea of walking for pleasure overlapped with the ebbing acceptance of walking for travel. Thomas West, an English priest, put pleasure walking into vogue in his guide to the Lake District of England published in 1778, "to encourage the taste of visiting the lakes by furnishing the traveller with a Guide; and for that purpose, the writer has here collected and laid before him, all the select stations and points of view, noticed by those authors who have last made the tour of the lakes, verified by his own repeated observations."

There was something about walking that people couldn't give up. We have been walking on two legs for eons and just forgetting about doing it rankles sensibility. But walking has never again been acceptable for travel, only as an activity or sport. After all, it's hard to go for a trip on foot, only a hike or adventure, neither of which involve traveling from one place to another, only out and back, unless someone is hiking the Appalachian or Pacific Crest

Trail. Then someone has to pick you up, probably in a car, at the end.

Today, travel on two feet has just recently become thought of in city design. Getting from one place to another on foot can be all but impossible, or at least treacherous. Walking some places is at best difficult and at worst dangerous because there are no sidewalks, paths, or crosswalks.   One of the most memorable descriptions of that state of affairs comes from Bill Bryon in his book *A Walk in the Woods* when he recounts his trip to Kmart to buy insect repellent. He made the trek on foot to the Kmart because he didn't have a car on his walk on the Appalachian Trail. The trip entailed walking on a busy road and falling down in the mud while trying to cross a creek under the highway because there was no way to cross the road. But, he found that Kmart was out of insect repellent.

It has begun to turn around. Health and city planning experts have discovered that having to use a car to get everywhere is neither good for health nor the environment. You wonder why it took so long since those factors have been obvious for decades. Today, a new mantra in city planning has become "walkability." Yes, it was all but impossible for Bill Bryson to get to the Kmart, and it still would be in many places. But city planners have begun to make cities more walkable by creating pedestrian- and bike-only areas so that people can go on foot to shop and congregate instead of by car.

Walkability refitting has created booming retail areas in places that had been suffering before. It has also made cities less polluted and healthier by not just cleaning the air but also getting people out on foot instead of cars.

Americawalks.org has come up with a list of principles for cities to become walkable.

- People of all abilities can safely walk and move along and across all streets in their communities.
- Communities of all sizes are designed so that most people can walk comfortably to places where they work, study, shop, play, and pray.
- States, counties, and cities revise existing transportation and development policies, standards, and programs to encourage walking, bicycling, and transit use.
- Transportation and development design decisions explicitly consider public health outcomes.

All that does make daily-life living in walkable areas more convenient for people who live there. What's missing for me is walking for pleasure, not for retail and restaurants, the big selling point for city planners. Some people do walk for pleasure on city streets and would not think of doing anything else. And good, it works for them. But to me, I look for solitude and nature to get the experience I crave, choose, and need for relaxation and work. I don't like to have to negotiate crowds and pay attention to people on sidewalks to get my walk in. Where people don't want to live in a densely populated area, crammed together, where zoning keeps retail and restaurants removed from residential areas, walkability is only a pipe dream. I live in such an area, but walking in nature and solitude is close at hand. In fact, as we will discuss in Chapter 5, "Ruminating Walking," walking in nature has a direct benefit for resetting the brain.

To achieve walkability, city planners have to make cities far more densely populated than they are now. So figure that as cities become more walkable, they will also get more and more people crammed into areas and nature farther away and less accessible.

There's a website where you can see how walkable your neighborhood is, walkscore.com. On their 0 to 100 scale, my neighborhood doesn't score too well with a "car dependent" score of 7, a "minimal transit" score of 16, and a "somewhat bikeable" score of 36. What they leave out is the "walking in nature" score, which I believe would be at least 80. And that, to me, anyway, is what's lacking in walkscore's walkability calculation, walking in nature. Yes, I would like to have stores more convenient, but I am grateful for how close nature is for my walks.

In spite of the new push for walkability, walkers mostly have been relegated. Places to walk in nature are carefully controlled, it seems. In order to walk there, we often have to drive. I much prefer to step out my front door to go for a walk. But we have come to expect that walking is an activity, not a mode of transportation, except in cities where walkability is valued. We harken back to the walkers who gloried in their walks, because in walking they were most creative, such as Socrates, Wordsworth, Rousseau, Nietzsche, and Thoreau who valued their walks as an opportunity to get their heads around a problem or even get their heads straight, something that was tolerated but maybe suspect. At least they weren't cluttering up the turnpikes but keeping to the woods and meadows.

Today we have "mall walkers," walking clubs, and even treadmills that make walking respectable because it is not to get somewhere but to get exercise or socialize. We'll look at contemplative walking, purposeful walking, joyful walking, meditative walking, ruminating walking, exploratory walking, and even "seeing if you can" walking later.

But enough of all that, I feel a walk coming on and I will be headed for nature.

Chapter 3
SEEING and Observing

'Tis very pregnant,

The jewel that we find, we stoop and take't

Because we see it; but what we do not see

We tread upon, and never think of it.

—William Shakespeare, "Measure for Measure" (Act II, Scene 1)

This morning on my walk I noticed a cholla (cactus) that I had never seen before. I know it has been there for at least a year since it is more than six feet tall. And it was not recently transplanted to that spot since you don't have to worry about a cholla growing; they come up unbidden, unaided by humans. It has become part of my consciousness and experience now. 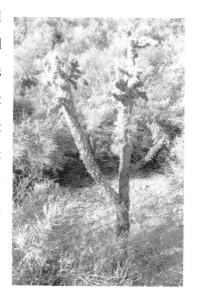 Is it important? Well, it is to me, and that's all that counts. It will stick with me until other things crowd it out of my mind and the cholla is packed up and stored in the old memory room under "nature," "cactus" and "walks" only to be unboxed when I relate it to some other knowledge or experience. It would be more fun to think about it having been transplanted, because then I could create an entire mental story about why and how. Unfortunately, what with showing its age and ailments, this cholla won't make it to the top ten of cactus beauty.

This chapter is about "seeing." What do we see, why do we see something, and how do we see it? Just noticing something doesn't qualify as "seeing," at least the way we're going to look at it here. Seeing things differently than we do now can provide a refreshing change to the experience of noticing the world and give walks a whole new dimension. This skill has come to me gradually. I cracked open the door and as I walked got the nerve to open it farther and farther. I have discovered an entire new world, one I had been missing because I was so intent on the walk itself, the distance, the number of steps. But it was there all the time sitting patiently for me to discover and enjoy it.

I have to wonder, is the wonderland the same for everyone when he or she cracks open the door and sees the new world, the new dimension awaiting discovery? I certainly don't know and have no way of finding out. All I can relate is my experience. It's like experiencing the glorious daybreak of the first morning, seeing what will become your favorite movie for the first time, becoming a poet without ever having to pen a single line, an explosion of beauty, of fascination, of wonder, of curiosity, of new horizons. Finally I wondered how I'd missed it all these years.

There's a difference between seeing and observing. We both see and observe to one degree or another all the time. There is a difference between everyday seeing and observing and ken seeing and observing. Observing is something we do to make better sense of the world around us. It can become a game to play with yourself or a friend. It can also make a walk much more interesting. Let's look at observing first.

Observing can be both useful and fun. Jack Foster in one of my favorite books *How to Get Ideas* writes about a game he used to play with his friend Bob Bean where they tested each other on their powers of observation. The first time they played the game, Foster asked his friend to put his head down and tell him, without looking, how many cash registers there were in the bar where they were sitting.

It got to be so much fun and so intoxicating (pun intended) that by the time "we stopped playing, there was nothing we didn't know." They observed such things as the names of "every bottle that's behind the bar," "what number was rung up on each cash register" when they walked in, and "how many chairs are there in here?" Did any of those facts matter? Matter to whom? In the overall scheme of things, I don't suppose they mattered at all, or maybe they did. They mattered to Jack and Bob, and that is all that matters, isn't it? It was the entertaining game they played.

Observing is often rewarded handsomely, celebrated in our world and in our literature. Just look at this example from Sherlock Holmes.

"When I hear you give your reasons," I [Dr. Watson] remarked, "the thing always appears to me to be so ridiculously simple that I could easily do it myself, though at each successive instance of your reasoning, I am baffled until you explain your process. And yet I believe that my eyes are as good as yours."

"Quite so," he [Holmes] answered, lighting a cigarette, and throwing himself down into an armchair. "You see, but you do not observe. The distinction is clear. For example, you have frequently seen the steps which lead up from the hall to this room."

"Frequently."

"How often?"

"Well, some hundreds of times."

"Then how many are there?"

"How many? I don't know."

"Quite so! You have not observed. And yet you have seen. That is just my point. Now, I know that there are seventeen steps, because I have both seen and observed."

--Arthur Conan Doyle, "A Scandal in Bohemia"

Then, how is "seeing" different from observing? Sir Arthur Conan Doyle (Holmes), uses "observing" the way I might describe "seeing." "Seeing" the number of steps is in line with more careful observation. I am sure there would be more to "see" with the steps. Some might be more worn than others; some might be worn on one side but not the other; then there's the nick out of the sixth step and the worn place on the tenth step that looks like an oak tree; and some might be different colors; and even more interestingly some might be plain old steps, whatever that is. Things we notice become significant only when we relate them to something we can relate to.

It isn't just the minutiae that we might "see," but also the macro observations such as, say, clouds and the look of trees, especially unusual trees such as the ghost tree pictured here. But as Shakespeare pointed out, "we see it, but what we 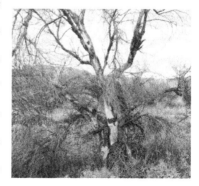 do not see we tread upon, and never think of it." "Seeing" enables us to think about it.

We can overcome this lack of observation "by cultivating the habit of watching things with an active, enquiring mind," writes O.E. Wilson. From there we have to decide how what we observe fits into our consciousness and experience. My natural curiosity makes that the fun part for me. What does that rock formation I just saw for the first time after having walked by it a dozen times at least, have to do with my experience in the world? Why did I just notice that today? Does it matter or is it just another item of interest? The importance and relevance of what we observe is our decision.

I am a fount of "useless" information; well, some people call it useless, anyway. I remember facts and figures, events and experiences, conversations and things I read that are of no particular use (at the time, anyway), like the cholla sitting unexpectedly next to the path. (I might be a terrific contestant in a pub trivia game depending on the questions, I suppose.) I am occasionally told that it might help if I remembered more important things, such as . . . oh, I don't remember, but it's surprising how often I can call on that "useless" information, and it sometimes helps.

But "seeing" can be the delight of the walk. Alexandra Horowitz in her fascinating book *On Looking* describes her observation as

For me, walking has become less physical transit than mental transportation. It is engaging. I have become, I fear, a difficult walking companion, liable to slow down and point at things. I can turn this off, but I love to have it on: a sense of wonder that I, and we all, have a predisposition to but have forgotten to enjoy.

We are all told to "pay attention." I heard that more times than I care to count from teachers. My mind wandered to places I would have rather been than where I was, trapped in the school room. There I was—finished, and the other kids were still poring over their work. My mind took me out the window to the world as I wished I was there instead of mentally chained to that chair in front of my desk. One year I often got to write notes to my parents saying how I should pay attention better. Trouble is, no one ever tells us how to pay attention. We must use our own system, whatever that is. It can be consciously observing or SEEING. Or, as Yogi Berra said, "You can observe a lot by watching."

SEEING with the vision of ken is different. We see the world differently, not better or worse, just differently. And the best part is that we can choose how we want to see the world either as observers or "seers," our own paying attention.

The shadows of the stones in the sunrise making new patterns.

I am not an expert in, nor an aficionado of, nor a practitioner of Zen. Rather I am looking for a different way of seeing things.

I can see no right or wrong way of experiencing the world. Instead, I am exploring ways to observe that take walking out of the realm of exercise and put it into one where exercise is incidental. The walk offers a new discovery or experience every time we step out our front doors. We can lose ourselves in the walk wandering outside the physical experience and letting our minds run free.

One of the most memorable descriptions I have come across for the experience of losing yourself in a walk is Bill Bryson's in his book *A Walk in the Woods*.

> But most of the time you don't think. No point. Instead, you exist in a kind of mobile Zen mode, your brain like a balloon tethered with string, accompanying but not actually part of the body below. Walking for hours and miles becomes as automatic, as unremarkable, as breathing. At the end of the day you don't think, 'Hey, I did sixteen miles today,' any more than you think, "Hey, I took eight-thousand breaths today." It's just what you do.

The true aficionados of Zen are more mystical than I am willing to get. I would rather stick to just experiencing things my own way, not necessarily the way we might have been conditioned to experience them or covering them up with earbuds playing an exercise playlist or Tony Robbins motivational recording. Nothing wrong with either of those, but they would interfere with my seeing and otherwise experiencing the world.

The best advice is "Do not think of anything" "Notice the light and how it hits certain objects and is blocked, causing shadows in others. Notice the quality and color of the light. Notice the shapes and lines of the objects and the natural, built in composition of the area. Use your other senses as well. Notice the aroma in the air. Feel the wind and listen to the ambient sounds." –Al Sanchez *the creator of PhotoTechniques.info, a site with digital photography tips*

He suggests using "your other senses as well." It all becomes part of the Zen experience that Bill Bryson mentions, "your brain like a balloon tethered with string, accompanying but not actually part of the body below."

How do we "not think of anything"? One way is to tell ourselves to "stop thinking." I have tried it on walks and found that it works up to a point. I stop thinking, at least for a while. At some point thoughts sneak back into my head and I may have less control over what those will be than I would prefer. After all, I have to watch where I'm going and stepping, so that requires a modicum of thought. Then I might "notice the light and how it hits certain objects," just as Al Sanchez suggests. I can also notice things like the ant craters that they build after it rains apparently to keep to water out of their ant holes. But I won't have had to stop thinking to notice them as I have on more than one occasion, watching the ants climb to the rim of the crater, stop, and turn around and go back to their hole. No idea why. It wasn't raining or wet, just cratered. It was fascinating. Stopping thinking definitely works in the middle of the night, even if not so well on a walk.

That's what we will give thought to in each chapter of this book, find what is fascinating during a walk, and maybe relate it to the SEEING experience.

The Night Chant

This prayer is part of a nine-day Navajo ritual called the Night Chant.

In beauty may I walk.

All day long may I walk.

Through the returning seasons may I walk.

Beautifully will I possess again.

Beautifully birds . . .

Beautifully joyful birds

On the trail marked with pollen may I walk.

With grasshoppers about my feet may I walk.

With dew about my feet may I walk.

With beauty may I walk.

With beauty before me, may I walk.

With beauty behind me, may I walk.

With beauty above me, may I walk.

With beauty below me, may I walk.

With beauty all around me, may I walk.

In old age wandering on a trail of beauty, lively, may I walk.

In old age wandering on a trail of beauty, living again, may I walk.

It is finished in beauty.

It is finished in beauty.

A Navajo Indian Prayer of the Second Day of the Night Chant (anonymous)

I feel a walk coming on with many new things to see and observe.

Chapter 4
Contemplative Walking

"We forget to wonder what we're missing as we hurry toward goals we may not even have chosen." Hannah Nyala, Point Last Seen

Before my walk one morning, I listened to the birds. Of course, the birds are up early every day to let us know it's time to get up. As soon as the first hint of light begins to push aside the night, the birds welcome the day. In the desert, it's always the "whit-wheet" of the Thrashers that starts it, sometimes followed shortly by the quail. Sometimes they trade off welcoming the day. No matter who starts it, though, it wakes you up in the morning, The birds keep at it all day. As I listened to the songs, I thought about using my senses when walking. Too often I use only one sense, sight. On my walk, I thought about it even more while I attuned to the different sounds I heard as I walked.

Along with Bob Marley's description, my world revealed itself;
Three little birds
Pitch by my doorstep
Singin' sweet songs
Of melodies pure and true

In addition to the birds, I heard traffic noise, in spite of the fact that I was nowhere near a major road until I reached the farthest outward point of my walk. Of course, it got louder and louder the nearer I got to the road where the traffic traveled 45 to 50 miles per hour. But there were other sounds besides the birds and the traffic. When I was on the dirt path, there was the sound of my footsteps.

Mostly I ignore them and am not conscious of footstep sounds where I walk because I expect to hear them. But that morning I thought about the different sounds that feet make as they strike the ground. On gravel, there's the crunch, crunch. As a boy, I remember listening to "dramas" on the radio. They added sound effects to simulate walking. It wasn't until years later that I learned how they made those sounds. There's also the skritch-skritch shoes make on the pavement when a stone gets stuck in the tread, and the squish-squish sound when walking through the mud, which I then have to clean off my shoes. If it's too bad, I leave them outside and clean them off later.

I hear different sounds when I walk on the sidewalk. My shoes are soft-soled, so they don't make much noise and sometimes what sound there is gets covered up by the ambient noise, a car going by, someone starting a car, a door closing. Even so, if I listen for them, I can hear anything from a swoosh-swoosh to a clop-clop depending on whether I am walking uphill or downhill.

When we walk contemplatively, we consciously use our senses. How often do we decide to use ignore every sense but one when we go for a walk? Taking advantage of just one makes it a different experience. We all experience the world with our senses differently, but we can decide how each time we walk. Will we "see" things, listen for the sounds, inhale the smells? It can be any or all of these.

As I said, I often default to sight only when I walk just so I can see things that I may not have seen before or notice things that had changed since the last time I walked by a spot, and of course, to keep from tripping. I ignore sounds, smell, touch, and taste, though, even if I decided to try it, touch and taste might be just a little difficult to pay attention to on a walk.

This morning I decided to experiment with touch for the first time. I made myself curious revising this chapter. Sight and sound are the easiest to focus on, but I wanted to experiment with how to use smell and touch. Smell? Not so good because my sense of smell is deficient. But touch I can do.

I'm almost never in a hurry, so I will take time to contemplate just about anything I fancy and touch requires stopping and feeling. The first thing I touched was palo verde bark. It's looks smooth but feels more like 60-grit sandpaper. Later in the walk, I touched another palo verde branch, and it was as smooth as it looked. But it was a young branch, not old enough to be grizzled.

Mesquite bark comes in all different varieties depending on the kind of mesquite. But all of it is every bit as rough as it looks— like a rough-hewn board only with more ridges and grooves. Live oak leaves look and feel like tiny saucers holding a drop or two of last night's rain

Never mind the cactus. It's all got thorns or other ways to impale you. Agave, though, is another story. It's a succulent for those of you who care, but it has smooth skin, even in the variety that can grow six o more feet tall. Well, it's smooth until you get to the edge of the stalk where there are finger-shredding spikes, or the point where it's ready to impale the unwary.

Desert Broom is a perfidious weed that is all but impossible to eradicate because its woody stalk grows up through the middle of other plants. The stalks with fine leaves don't feel like leaves but just rough places. One aside is that desert broom's seeds look like smoke blowing around.

But since sight is a fun sense to use, so on many walks, I look for new sights. It could be something I have "seen" already, but not seen such as the cholla in Chapter 2. Then there was the day I saw the fat buds of a palo verde tree. I don't know how I had missed them before because they were hanging at eye level over the street, right there for me to walk into. I'm rarely in a hurry when I walk and I wasn't that morning, so I stood and stared at them for a while, firmly etching them in my brain. I can still see them now as I call them up. They will stay with me until they are boxed up and stored in the old memory room.

Another morning I noticed the water meter for a house at street level with the house sitting up at least 20 feet above the street. With my fascination for contemplating the odd, I wondered if they had to have a pump to get enough water pressure to service the house. Then when I looked behind me, I could see how far downhill I had walked and figured the speed of the water in the pipe would be plenty powerful enough to make it up to the house's level.

Different people experience walking in the world differently depending on their predilections and their size. Alexandra Horowitz in one chapter of her excellent book *On Looking: A Walker's Guide to the Art of Observation*, in one of my favorite passages, describes accompanying her 19-month-old son, as "about not walking." It describes how to experience the world anew, oh, so devoutly to be wished. Her son turned what we might describe as just a walk as a new experience every time he sets foot out the door with his mother.

"It has nothing to do with points, A, B, or getting from one to the other. A walk is, instead, an investigatory exercise that begins with energy and ends when (and only when) exhausted. "

She continues, describing the "walk" as an exploration for a 19-month-old, "exploring surfaces and textures with finger, toe, and—yuck—tongue [touch and taste]." And observation, "standing still and seeing who or what comes by, ' then there's adventure, "trying out different forms of locomotion (among them running, marching, high-kicking, galloping, scooting, projectile falling, spinning, and noise shuffling)."

A "walk" is also an investigation. There's the "discarded candy wrapper; collecting a fistful of pebbles and a twig and a torn corner of a paperback; swishing dirt back and forth along the ground." And finally, there's sound, "the murmuring of the breeze in the trees; locating the source of a bird's song;"

I can only imagine what "projectile falling" is and most likely don't care to try. But a 19-month-old sees, hears, and senses so many things that we simply don't see, hear, or otherwise sense. After all, it's old hat and unworthy of our notice. Walking contemplatively we also have the opportunity to see, hear, touch, and otherwise sense the world from a perspective far different than that of a 30-inch tall person. By taking ourselves back to what we imagine the world was like when we were 19 months old, every walk can be a new and exciting experience. I'm going to work on it. And unlike my exploration of a state highway when I was 18 month old, I will make a point of remembering these walks.

Others experience the world differently. One morning as I was wandering back toward home on my walk, a young man turned a corner in front of me wearing headphones. Presumably, the headphones were attached to an iPod or Smartphone and playing music, an audio recording of a book, or motivational message. I, of course, have no way of knowing which. Whatever he was listening to, it most likely works for him. I also often see another young man walking his German Shepherd. He doesn't have headphones on, but is moving right along behind his "walk-ecstatic dog," arm stretched to its limit, shoulder nearly dislocated (it's a big dog), unsuccessfully trying to pull the dog back to a more comfortable pace, per Harold Monro's enticing poem, "Dog."

> We are going OUT. You know the pitch of the word,
> Probing the tone of thought as it comes through fog
> And reaches by devious means (half-smelt, half-heard)
> The four-legged brain of a walk-ecstatic dog.

I often see other people walking and wearing, and presumably listening with, ear buds. These aren't kids, but mature adults who are maybe using their walk to listen to an audio book or motivational recording, but often as I pass them, I hear the music. Online music services offer playlists for all kinds of activities, making the sounds they choose to hear and enjoy assist them in their activity. Amazon even has playlists "Walking the Dog" and "Hip Hop for Walking." It could be an effective use of time.

While it's not what I would choose to do, I understand completely. I simply prefer nature and the world around me as I contemplate my walking experience.

My point is this. Sounds surround us that we rarely hear because we don't listen for them. That morning I mesmerized myself listening for them. Obviously, the young man with the headphones was listening to his own sounds, not those of the world surrounding him. Those listening to audio books while they walk are rewarded. That is, of course, their choice and not my business why. It's simply a matter of interest. The young man walking his dog was also experiencing the world with at least one different sense, the dog pulling hard on the leash stretching his shoulder.

How can we sense the world like a 19-month-old? How can we begin to see it freshly each time we venture out into the world? What can we do to put a new light on what is around us all the time?

The OED (Oxford English Dictionary) provides a couple of appropriate definitions of contemplative: "Given to or having the habit of contemplation; meditative, reflective, thoughtful." And "Looking or gazing at." I prefer to add contemplative walking means to me sensing the world around me and thinking about what I see, hear, smell, touch, feel, or taste, not just gaze or look at. And since this is my book, I guess I can make it mean anything I want because that's what I want it to mean. Kind of like Humpty Dumpty, "'When I use a word,' Humpty Dumpty said in rather a scornful tone, 'it means just what I choose it to mean — neither more nor less.' [So **mine** is just a **tiny** stretch of definition.]

"'The question is,' said Alice, 'whether you can make words mean so many different things.'

'The question is,' said Humpty Dumpty, 'which is to be master — that's all."

We are all masters of how we perceive our environments and what they mean. When we walk alone, as William Hazlitt writes, we decide what we will contemplate and what that will mean to us.

One of the pleasantest things in the world is going a journey; but I like to go by myself. I can enjoy society in a room; but out of doors, nature is company enough for me. I am then never less alone than when alone. –William Hazlitt

I feel a walk coming on. What sense will I use today?

Chapter 5
Ruminating Walking

Have brain fog? Easily distracted? Worry shutting off effective work? Yeah, me too. It's a virus that attacks randomly, it seems, and often at the most inopportune times, the times when I most need my brain working at top speed and clarity. All is not lost. I've found a way to at least make it better and maybe all well. Here's how I kill the virus and restore my dwindling focus and clarity—walking along and in nature.

You see, I need unfettered time to sort out whatever it is I am trying to sort, an editing problem, an article idea, a book chapter, or just my foul mood. The trick is the unfettering. Being in motion is the key, but not just any motion. The motion must be away from city streets and people, or the even more distracting treadmill in a fitness center with 10 TVs showing depressing, mind-sucking news. In nature and alone.

Sure, walking gets blood flowing, usually to the brain no matter where the walking takes place, and that helps thinking, but there's something called Directed Attention Fatigue that gets in the way of the brain doing a proper job. It gets in the way because our brains get overloaded with detritus that interfere with our ability to direct our attention where we had in mind in our fog. More about that and about the study that showed how it works in a minute.

I ruminate a lot, and I need to be clear and focused if I'm going to get anything out of it. Some people talk things out. Some people need other people to bounce ideas off of. It works for them but not for me. I think things out. I ruminate. I assemble information and then let it filter through my brain, regurgitate maybe with a different slant, work itself around to become a complete thought (still needing more rumination), and find its way into proper opening, maybe becoming something I can use. But my surroundings have a lot to do with how well rumination works.

Too much stress, too much distraction, too much energy sapping and instead of percolating, it's Swiss cheese. Where percolation sends ideas through tiny holes where they find their appropriate places, with Swiss cheese, thoughts don't even slow down. They zoom on through the big holes and lose themselves in more detritus, sometimes never to be heard from again.

I think better, well maybe at all, when both alone and in nature. I lose focus as soon as I get where people, traffic and myriad distractions interfere. I have to acknowledge people even if only to nod or wave at people and watch out for traffic and people with dogs. It turns out I am not weird at least in that way. It's an actual affliction and normal, not just me. A 2008 study at the University of Michigan by Marc Berman, et al, compared two groups. One group of students Berman had walk in nature. The other on city streets in Ann Arbor, Michigan. gave them a backward digit span task after they finished. This is a test to see how many numbers someone can remember both backward and sometimes forward. The group that walked in nature did far better than did the city-street walkers.

Then, just in case the result was unique to the group itself, they switched sides. The city-streets group walked in nature while the nature group walked on city streets. Same results. The nature group did better on the backward digit span task. Just as interesting, they redid the study in the winter with the frigid, snowy weather in Ann Arbor. They had one group trudge through the snow in nature while the other group walked on possibly icy city streets. Then they switched them again. Same result. Weather conditions didn't matter. Walking in nature had a decided benefit in the ability to concentrate.

This study followed several others that had discovered the same thing. It has to do with a phenomenon called Attention Restoration Theory that shows that "directed attention" is restored by interaction with nature. Being over-stimulated by internal and external stimuli results in Directed Attention Fatigue, which means being more distractible, having trouble listening, hearing things wrong, or missing things. In addition, people may have trouble focusing, leave things half done, forget things, lose things, find it hard to think, get confused more easily, think less creatively. Or they may get stuck on certain ideas, thoughts. In other words, their "cognitive control" is affected negatively. Study.com offered this definition of cognitive control: "your mind's ability to actively create an information picture that will guide your behavior. It's what allows you to select a certain behavior that you have accepted as appropriate and reject a behavior that you have decided is inappropriate." We'll dig into "internal stimuli" in the "Mindful Meditation Walking" chapter—up next in Chapter 6.

"In every walk with nature, one receives far more than he seeks."—John Muir

As the 2008 study concluded, they showed "that simple and brief interactions with nature can produce marked increases in cognitive control," thus restoring directed attention. Just how simple and brief? They don't say. I suppose you just have to go for walks in nature to see what works. There is no right or wrong in walking, only what is effective for each person. In Chapter 7, we'll look at just how inaccurate many of those mantras about recommended amounts of exercise are.

Resetting directed attention by walking in nature is the key, though. If I am going to work even remotely effectively, my ability to direct attention must be focused, not short circuited by chaos or over-stimulation by having to deal with other people, people's dogs, and traffic. My attention needs restoring. It doesn't require much distraction to defocus my attention and muddle my ability to put ideas into some a modicum of workable form.

Just as good, every walk is a discovery process. Some days I come up with pages of ideas. Other days I don't think of anything. I just enjoy the walk. In her autobiography, the French writer Sidonie-Gabrielle Colette wrote, "There are days when solitude is heady wine that intoxicates you, others when it is a bitter tonic, and still others when it is a poison that makes you beat your head against the wall." Huh, so I am not unique.

Rarely do I resort to head beating; in fact I can't remember the last time. Going for a walk isn't a punishment, a sentence that must be endured, such as the "taking of medicine" Thoreau mentioned in Chapter 1. It is both a pleasure and an opportunity to get ideas. But ideas alone are insufficient. I know lots of ways to come up with ideas. Some of them actually work. Some work sometimes, but none of them works every time. The trouble is, ideas are a penny apiece and that's all they're worth until we make them worth pursuing, flesh them out, create a plan to put them into practice, and a foolproof way to make them successful. None of that happens for me if my attention is constantly disrupted.

How do I flesh out ideas? One way is the mindstorming method. I first heard about mindstorming on a tape series by Brian Tracy. His website even now provides complete instructions for it. It's a nifty approach, but requires solitude. As he described it, you get a blank sheet of paper, you turn off your phone, you don't answer the door, you have sufficient writing instruments so you don't have to stop if a pen runs out of ink or a pencil lead breaks, you write a question at the top of the page, and you think of 20 ways to answer that question. I don't think this process would work on a smart phone, but what do I know.

As in brainstorming, you switch off criticism and just write whatever ideas come to mind. The trick is, you don't stop until you have written 20 answers. Most people will not sit still that long, but it pays off if done to completion. As Brian Tracy describes it, the first five or 10 come easily. Then it gets harder. By the time you get to 17, 18, 19, and 20, the ideas become extraordinarily useful and productive. No need to worry as you write them down if they are any good. You can always go back, be critical, and scratch out the mundane or stupid ideas, after all. For example, this chapter has been the most difficult for me to organize. Maybe I didn't have enough alone time or I got distracted on my walks or I had other things to think about. The 20 ideas plan may not work while walking alone, but the ideas often come even though as Ms. Colette pointed out, it is "sometimes bitter tonic." That's okay. I have learned not to force it because ideas can't be forced. They can only flow when they are developed enough to flow. Ideas will come as they are willing but not before my brain fog is banished along with Directed Attention Fatigue.

When they do come and I have recovered, I may have lots to work on, or maybe just enough.

Keeping the ideas that I have come up with is essential. I have tried different idea memory tricks, ways to keep my ideas safe and easily retrievable to flesh out and create plans for. Recording them on my phone as I thought of them kind of worked, but I cast that one aside. Writing them down works much better for me. I carry a notebook just for that purpose. The advantage of a notebook is that writing the idea often generates more ideas because I not only write it kinesthetically but also see it. Along with 60 percent of the population, I am a visual learner, so seeing helps me not only remember but also gives me a springboard for ways to make the ideas work. Other people may find that a voice recorder works best for them. There is no right or wrong way to keep thoughts straight. My learning style is why I use pen and paper.

I find that the additional advantage is the record in the notebook of what I thought about. Going back through the pages of notes I have taken, I can often come up with even more ideas days and weeks later. When I get back from my walk sometimes the creative juices have flowed to the extent that I have an entire article or chapter worked out. I can sit down, refer to my notes, and create the beginnings of a masterpiece, or at least something acceptable that I can probably fix.

As to mind storming while walking, I have tried it and it doesn't work well for me. However, when I get back from a walk, it does work. After all, my directed attention is restored, so I have had my ability to focus restored along with my ability to think an idea through. It is walking that gets the brain going. I'll look at the physical reason for that in Chapter 7. And there's something about walking in nature, alone that gets it going even more, at least for me. I can't speak for anyone else because we don't all walk to get ideas. It may be to socialize, to exercise, to see sights, even busy city sights, or follow a tour group with a tour guide. But I walk to get ideas, to work, to get over "Directed Attention Fatigue."

The Reverse Option

It turns out we might have been walking in or at least facing the wrong direction. I was turned on to an article by Dr. Joseph Mercola in which he cited two studies that show walking backwards can "enhance cognitive control."

Two studies examined the effects of walking backwards. A 2009 study from Radboud University Nijmegen in the Netherlands by Severine Koch and others found that if we walk backwards, we may enhance our capability to deal with a difficult situation by mobilizing "cognitive resources." All they had their test subjects do was walk four steps in each direction and give Stroop tasks to each. A Stroop task is where say one color of ink is used but the word printed in the color is another, for example, the color red might say green. Walking backwards made a significant difference in how well people were able to identify the correct word.

Aleksandar Aksentijevic and others followed up that study in 2018 with another in the United Kingdom by where they did memory tests after their test subjects had walked backwards like the tests at the University of Michigan I mentioned earlier.

The results showed that walking backwards increased the test subjects' abilities to remember both a crime scene video and a memory questionnaire. The increased memory lasted about 10 minutes, they found. In this study, they had the test subjects walk backwards for 10 meters, about 33 feet.

Of course, I had to try it. On my walk this morning, I walked backwards for 50 steps, that's at least 33 feet, on three different occasions, carefully of course, and in nature, so got double advantage. I didn't have a memory test to give myself, but wanted to see what would happen. Having gotten off on one of its usual tangents that had nothing to do with what I wanted to work on; describing exactly what did happen escapes me, but things seemed a little clearer and sharper and my brain began working on this chapter again. The true test will be to see if it continues to work and what walking backwards does exactly.

This system, well these systems both walking in nature and backwards, most likely work best for people who want to use walks to get ideas, to sort out issues, to think things through, or anything else that requires directed attention. As Christopher Long and James Averill wrote in their study "Solitude: An Exploration of Benefits of Being Alone,"

> Creativity consists of forming associations between previously unrelated ideas and giving expression to those associations in ways that are useful or valuable to the self or others. We consider here two ways in which solitude can facilitate creativity—first, by stimulating imaginative involvement in multiple realities and, second, by "trying on" alternative identities, leading, perhaps, to self-transformation. These, and creativity more generally, could not occur without a loosening—deconstruction and subsequent reconstruction—of cognitive structures.

I can't and won't prescribe any particular reason or method for going for a walk. This one works for me. People walk for their own reasons and in their own environments. For me, ruminating is worthwhile, productive, and a joy and best done in nature.

"Never did I think so much, exist so much, be myself so much as in the journeys I have made alone and on foot. Walking has something about it which animates and enlivens my ideas. I can

hardly think while I am still; my body must be in motion to move my mind." – Jean-Jacques Rousseau

I feel a walk coming on.

Chapter 6
Mindful Meditation Walking

1-2-3-4-5-6-7-8-9-10 counting steps. Breathe in two steps, and breathe out two steps. Those are two ways to begin to walk meditatively with the goal walking "mindfully." Mindfulness, says dictionary.com is "a technique in which one focuses one's full attention only on the present, experiencing thoughts, feelings, and sensations but not judging them."

Lao Tzu summed it up, "If you're depressed, you're living the in past. If you're anxious, you're living in the future. But if you're at peace, you're living in the moment." Meditation and attaining mindfulness, either sitting still or walking, aim to put yourself at peace. I had to try it. After all, this book is about my experiences walking, so if I didn't try it out, how could I explain it?

I can attest to Mark Twain's observation, "I've had a lot of worries in my life, most of which never happened." Mark Williams and Danny Penman wrote in their book *Mindfulness* that our thoughts should be our servants rather than our masters. They suggested that thoughts are just events in the mind and not reality. They wrote, "We re-live past events and re-feel their pain, and we pre-live future disasters and so pre-feel their impact." Mark Twain knew and I know exactly what they mean. I can dredge up past negative events and just get more and more angry and irritated.

Then I can switch over to thinking about something that might happen even six months from now and get equally worked up. Wow! That does a lot of good, doesn't it? In the meantime, the productive thing I could have been working on or thinking about sits idle, waiting patiently for me to get over my irritation and obsession about some past harm or slight or sort out how I will deal with a mythical future event that most likely will never happen, or of course, will happen, just watch.

One bi-product of living in the past and the future is that everything has to be judged. Meditative/mindfulness walking is supposed to turn that off. We can just observe. "My, isn't that interesting." "Just look at how he did that." "I always have admired that color car." "I wonder what that vanity license plate means?" "That guy must have had an important place to be to drive that fast and run that red light." Things, past, present, and future, become items of interest rather than things I have to pass judgment on. Also appropriate are the things I looked at in the Contemplative Walking chapter, listen to the sound my feet make on the ground, listen to the birds, notice something new on my walk, or smell the odor of whatever nature or feel the bark of a tree when I walk by.

My brain always works at least at 6,752 miles per hour. Does it need to slow down? I suffer sometimes from the "directed attention fatigue" I wrote about in the ruminating chapter. Would walking mindfully, meditating while walking, slowing down help reverse that problem in addition to the walking in nature solution? I read all the material I could find about how to do it and about all the benefits. It turns out there are additional benefits besides just the shutting off of negative thoughts, but I'll get into that in a bit.

Alan Castel wrote in his article, "Why Should We Slow Down? The Lost Art of Patience," that "slowing down can make you more aware of the dangers of walking and falling." He points out that the average American "checks his or her smart phone once every six-and-a-half minutes, or roughly 150 times a day." It's no wonder that people wander off into the street intently looking at their phones and ignoring the bus bearing down on them. He adds that "there is something to be gained by being slow if slow can make you more present, more mindful, and more aware of other people's perspectives." I know I try to slow down both my brain and walking speed when I walk because, other than the enjoyment of the walk, I walk so I can work, so I can get ideas, so I can get my head around issues I need to deal with, either pleasant or not so. To write in my notebook, I have to stop entirely for a minute. If I don't, I will have even less of a chance to read my own writing when I try to decipher it later.

And that leads to the caveat about paying attention while walking. We have to pay attention to where we are walking and possible hazards that could result in ruining a perfectly good walk and possible an entire day or month, or maybe a forever. Sitting meditation, the usual method, only involves maybe putting oneself partially in touch with the world. That works while walking about as well as checking your phone while you are crossing the street paying no attention to the approaching bus.

I didn't know anything about walking meditatively and being mindful before I began researching this chapter. Even though I have meditated sitting or lying down, almost immediately falling asleep if I am lying down, I had no idea about how to go about walking meditatively. I set out to investigate. It turns out the information about it is considerable. I tried to get information about mindful walking from supposed experts and practitioners, but none of the 20 or so people I called or email bothered to even respond to my questions and offers to interview them for this book.

The instructions I found in books and on websites differ mostly in how complicated they make the meditative walk. I prefer simple, so that's what I went for. If you want more complicated, by all means do a search on the internet. You will come up with a plethora of ways to walk mindfully that involve convoluted preparation, requiring 10 to 15 minutes of preparation before I set one foot out the door. No, I don't have time for that. I want to go for a walk.

Mostly, I want to know if mindful meditative walking would benefit me. If it would, how? And how might I describe or define a benefit?

I read seemingly all the material; then I was eager to see if mindful meditative walking would help. I started out counting steps from one to 10 and then starting over again. Then I tried the more complicated counting, 1, 1-2, 1-2-3, 1-2-3-4, . . . 1-2-3-4-5-6-7-8-9-10. and then started over. But it is more than just step counting. Counting steps must be done with intention. That means walking probably more slowly than regular walking speech, consciously thinking about each step. Believe me, it's easy to count steps unconsciously and still have my brain go off on flights of re-living and pre-living.

Did it work? Having forgotten where I was, sometimes I had to just continue from where I thought I had left off. I am able to get through the entire count without losing my place now. The thing I have noticed is that it does allow me to think and be in the present even if that involves thinking about which foot ends up where in the count for each number of steps. I don't know if that is a desired effect, but it does make from re-living the past and pre-living the future all but impossible.

Then there is the counting breaths method. One website suggests one breath in per step and one breath out per step. I tried it and it's way too slow, not even walking. I just stepped. I am going for a walk, not a step. I remembered that when I ran, oh so many years ago, I would breathe in for a count of four and breathe out for a count of two. I don't use as much oxygen walking as I did running, so that didn't work. But if I breathed in for a count of two steps and out for a count of two, that worked and doesn't slow me down any. It works going uphill and downhill, but I don't always think about it or use it. Walking at a normal pace on a flat surface requires only unconscious breathing.

The result has been encouraging. When I start out my walk by counting steps or breaths, I find that after five or 10 minutes, I am often able to generate ideas such as those I discussed in the ruminating walking chapter far more frequently and for a longer time than I had been if I just chugged off down the street. That's another benefit. Because, after all, I work when I walk, so anything that helps me focus benefits me and my work.

The key, as Padmapreetham Mahalingam pointed out on the website boldsky.com, is "to set the intention that walking is for the purpose of meditation." He also observed that mindful walking allows "you to enjoy the pleasure of walking." My experience backs that up—so far.

So what happened when I tried these different methods? All three, counting steps two ways and counting breaths, turned off my re-living and pre-living and allowed me at least sometimes for a minute or two to be in the present. Other times the negative spiral persisted, hanging on as a spiteful obsession no matter how much I tried to get rid of it. I was warned that we have to do it for 15 or 20 minutes for full effect. Trouble was, at first I was done after two or three minutes and without my desired effect. As I practiced it, though, I worked up to five minutes. Five minutes was better than three minutes, but didn't have the complete desired effect, or what I imagined was the complete desired effect. Now on many walks, I start out counting steps or breaths and am getting better. If I stop because I need to concentrate on where I am going or something I see, I can start up again when I get to a place that doesn't require physical attention such as traffic, trip hazards, and dogs.

It does work, Mindful meditative walking has benefits. It resets my brain in a way that lets me focus on what I want to focus on rather than spiraling into the past or obsessing about the future.

The technique that works for me, at least most of the time, is to walk meditatively on smooth, even surfaces rather than on uneven, rocky, potholed areas. If I want to meditate some in the uneven areas, I find a quiet, unpopulated place to sit. The extra, added advantage of mindful meditation is that you are aware of the world around you instead of possibly meditating a different way and drifting off into the ether somewhere. Different ways work better sitting, but are not safe while walking.

The other benefit of all kinds of meditation is that it promotes stress reduction because it "improved both physical and emotional responses to stress," reports WebMD in an article on its website. In addition, it is purported in several studies to not only reduce stress, but to boost immune functioning, reduce chronic pain, and lower blood pressure. Several studies I have read discovered why that works, but I won't go into them here since I cannot personally attest to their improving responses to stress. Just do a search for studies on meditation on the internet, if you are interested and see if it works for you.

All those meditative mindful walking techniques I found work for me, and I have found that becoming mindful when I walk helps me focus on the work I need to do, sometimes with pages of ideas but other times only with a pleasant walk. I feel a walk coming on.

Chapter 7
Seniors Walking

Some people are old while they are still young. Some people don't realize they're old. Still other people never get old. That one can be either a plus or minus. The minus is dying before they reach the age that qualifies as old. The plus is staying so active that old age never catches up. That's what I want to do.

And that's the trick, isn't it? Trouble is, I can't do all the things I could do 30 and 40 years ago and recover from them in a day or so. In fact, I can't do all the things I could do 20 years ago and get over them quickly. Truth be told, I can't even approach doing some of the things I could do 20, 30, or 40 years ago no matter what. I need to correct that. There's that annoying stiffness. Mind you, I've never been particularly flexible. For example, I have never been able to touch my toes without bending me knees. But more about stiffness later.

I qualify in age as a senior but miss qualifying completely with my physical condition. According to the National Council on Aging, "Approximately 80% of older adults have at least one chronic disease, and 77% have at least two. Four chronic diseases—heart disease, cancer, stroke, and diabetes—cause almost two-thirds of all deaths each year." I am fortunate in that I don't have any of those. Old age is hot on my tail but running out of breath and I haven't, at least so far.

I walk about 25 miles a week, usually a little more, occasionally less, but outpacing old age isn't the reason. It's for other benefits. I work when I walk. I also enjoy my surroundings and glory in the sounds I hear, the experiences I have, the surprises I see, and the new places I explore.

So how much should I be walking to keep outrunning, or outwalking, old age? Those who claim to know have created formulae and standards, without any basis in scientific evidence. Somewhere, sometime, someone came up with the "magic" number of 30 minutes a day, five days a week for walking to maintain health. I asked experts, trainers, and therapists and spent hours looking for the study that proved that, but as far as I can determine, it doesn't exist. The first mention of that number came with the 1991 Department of Health and Human Services publication *Healthy People 2000*. They posited the 30 minutes a day number (first on page 73 then repeated as gospel three times). However, they cite no study, peer reviewed or otherwise, to prove that number is ideal, enough, or too much. All they said was that people don't get enough exercise. Well, duh, and then threw out the number of 30 minutes a day. Certainly it most likely can't hurt, but so what? Even so, 30 minutes a day, five days a week is parroted and become gospel in almost every instance where exercise amount is suggested for "older" people, and, as it happens, just about everyone.

As I told a doctor who suggested that to me, I'll never get any tougher if that's all I do. It only maintains current condition and doesn't make me stronger. For many people 30 minutes may be the maximum of their physical ability while for others, such as myself, it's barely a warm-up. As we get stronger and more physically fit, the minimum can actually result in our physical condition deteriorating. My intention is to get stronger and stronger, always gaining on the relentlessly pursuing gremlin of old age.

Then there's the 10,000 steps mantra. That was made up out of whole cloth by a Japanese company before the 1964 Tokyo Olympics. One Dr. Yoshiro Hatano began selling a 10,000 step pedometer known as "manpo-kei" (translation: 10,000 steps meter). He had found that the average Japanese walked 3,500 to 5,000 steps a day. He calculated that if someone walked 10,000 steps a day, it could burn up 20 percent of a person's daily calories. Well maybe, but that reasoning is circular because the evidence is "proved" by the conclusion. The magic number was to sell pedometers. But so what? If the goal is just better health, that's one thing. If it's to lose weight, it doesn't come close to losing a pound.

Different people have different physical conditions and 10,000 steps can be walked in different terrains. Certainly 10,000 steps at the mall burns up far fewer calories than does 10,000 steps climbing hills. Moreover, walking doesn't burn many calories. Walking one hour on a level surface burns 270 calories in an hour. Walk an hour over a 2 percent grade and the total goes up to 307 calories. Walking 10,000 steps is supposed to burn up 20 percent of daily calories. The only way to come close to understanding what Hatano was getting at is to add 20 percent to calorie usage. Thus, over the 270 calories in an hour, we add 54 calories and over 307 we add 61 calories. To lose a pound, it requires burning 3500 calories. Walking the "recommended" 30 minutes a day, five days a week, burns 675 calories or 768 calories walking 10,000 steps. The walking 10,000 steps helps, of course, to make someone feel better, feel a sense of accomplishment, and get blood moving, but doesn't make much difference in weight. Regardless, those 10,000 steps have become a mantra.

One of the biggest fears for seniors is "losing it." Some days I could swear I am. But walking helps brain health and I at least think I think better after a walk. Recent scientific studies tossed that 10,000 step mantra into the rubbish heap of nonsense, at least for brain health. A study at the UCLA Semel Institute for Neuroscience and Human Behavior found that 4,000 steps is enough to help brain health. Those findings were published in the *Journal of Alzheimer's Disease.* Each member of the study group had complained of memory problems at the beginning of the study.

The researchers did an MRI to determine the thickness of the hippocampus, the room in the brain where memory is stored. Hippocampus thickness is a predictor of how effective memory will be. The study found that people who walked more than 4,000 steps a day had thicker hippocampi and related brain regions than did those who walked fewer steps. I don't know why the study used the cutoff of 4,000 steps. Would 3,500 have been just about as effective? Maybe 5,000 would have done an even better job. The researchers have yet to do a longitudinal study to find out if walking 4,000-plus steps a day continues to keep memory intact.

The reason for the increased memory and probably brain function was shown in a study conducted by New Mexico Highlands University. The study mostly "concentrated on running's effects on carotid artery blood flow as a result of heel impact." They found that foot strike exercise—both walking and running—pushes more blood to the brain and that helps our brains work better. Dr. Ernest Greene, first author of the study, said, "What is surprising is that it took so long for us to finally measure these obvious hydraulic effects on cerebral blood flow. There is an optimizing rhythm between brain blood flow and ambulating." Translated that means running and walking sends more blood to the brain.

I knew there had to be a reason I worked better, enjoyed my surroundings more, and felt better when I walked. Think how much less fulfilling a walk would be if it took blood away from the brain and sent it to our legs, hands, or fingers, or just had it sit there flowing where it had been. My rewarding experience would vanish into a cloud of guilt and frustration. (more about guilt in Chapter 14.

Another thing we almost always see in articles about getting into an exercise program is to check with your doctor. In a 1995 article in the Journal of the American Medical Association, "Physical Activity and Public Health," the authors say "Most adults do not need to see their physician before starting a moderate-intensity physical activity program." So unless someone has a chronic disease or plans to jump into a "vigorous" program, "Just Do It," as Nike ads used to say.

With all this plucked-from-the-air data trying to tell me what to do, how much physical activity do I need to aim at? For me, it's whatever makes me feel good, proud of myself, and gets my blood moving. I wouldn't presume to tell anyone how much activity he or she should get. Even if I knew what that person's condition was, I still wouldn't suggest anything. It's up to the individual. We are all adults and capable of making our own decisions about what works for us. Thus, if a certain amount of exercise works for someone, that's most likely appropriate using whatever criteria that person believes is appropriate. We'll look at the physical health benefits of walking in Chapter 15 and how to measure heart rate and appropriate exercise intensity subjectively.

Then there's the stiffness.

Many years ago I knew Norm. He and his wife owned a ballroom dance studio, and of course, both were not only experienced but dedicated dancers. Norm was over six feet tall and over 70 years old when I knew him. I often see "older" men inching their ways out of cars and walking stooped over, with tentative steps and stiff hips.. Norm had no sign of that. After all, he was a dancer. His biggest enjoyment in life was dancing, if not with his wife Helen, then with any other woman who would dance with him. He could dance a 35 year old off the dance floor.

I didn't think anything about how Norm was limber and walked like a young man, but I thought of him today. He didn't stiffen up as he got older because he danced every chance he got. I want to be like Norm, not a dancer but limber walking like a young man as I age. So I guess if someone doesn't like walking much but truly enjoys dancing, it's just as good at keeping or getting oneself lithe and limber.

Jon Burras of jonburras.com posits something that I particularly like and am eager to agree with even if I question it. We are often told that we can expect to stiffen up as we age, but Burras disagrees. He says that it is stiffness that causes aging, not the other way around. He argues in one document that "If aging were responsible for the hardening and stiffening of your body then *everyone* who is alive or who has ever lived would have a hardened and tight body." Instead, it is the fact that we stop moving our bodies and let emotions take over our muscles. He is a yoga practitioner and says that one thing that will help stiffness and fend off "old age" is Expansive Movement. Expansive Movement practices will "energize and liquefy the body tissues and not harden and stiffen them." He warns against the desiccation of muscles that happens when we allow them to stiffen up and advocates putting the fluid that we had when we were younger back in them. Of course, some people have been stiff their entire lives, but everyone can benefit by working on loosening up their bodies and be like Norm or Jon.

Burras says that most people don't spend enough time stretching. I know that fits my predilections. I sometimes stretch before I walk, but only briefly. I want to get at it. Stretching helps me to enjoy a walk more than if I just whiz out the door. I almost never stretch when I am finished with my walk, and that is just as or even more important, Burras says. "This is often the missing link in our health and wellness." I know from personal experience that it feels wonderful to stretch. My entire body loosens up. Any muscle soreness either disappears or eases at least a bit. When I finish working with my personal trainer every week, the last thing he has me do is spend a few minutes stretching the muscles he has tortured. It feels better then.

All that sounds good, but I want to know why I get stiff sometimes, and I'm far from certain that Burras is correct. He provides no scientific evidence nor does he cite any studies, peer reviewed or otherwise, to back up his claim.

What I found interesting in my stiffness research is its relationship to inflammation. Paul Ingraham, a science writer and former massage therapist from Vancouver, British Columbia, writes that "by far the most familiar sources of inflammation –and stiffness—is probably aging. Everyone gets more inflamed as they age." He calls it inflammaging, and that is "a set of biological dysfunctions strongly linked to poor fitness, obesity, aging, and likely emotional stress and sleep disturbances, as well." But that reasoning, just like the 10,000 steps goes around in circles. We have stiffness because we are inflamed and we are inflamed because we are stiff. Which came first? Which one caused the other? Years don't necessarily make you stiff because it's an individual situation. So I looked further into it.

We get inflamed for any number of reasons, so the trick is to de-inflame or avoid inflammation whenever possible. There are the anti-inflammatory foods that you can look up yourself numerous places, and foods and drinks that don't cause inflammation and much of that is unique to the individual. There is also having your body become too acidic. The solutions for that are readily available too, and some I take advantage of sometimes. The "old age condition" can result in inflammation because our livers can't process the things that make us inflamed as quickly, and so they get stuck in our bodies as they didn't when we were in our 20s and 30s, and maybe even 40s.

All this discussion about the proper number of steps can make someone feel like a failure if he or she doesn't "measure up" to some artificial standard.

The number of steps has become a game for me. I keep track of steps and add them up at the end of the week to see how I have done. Walking 25 miles, about 50,000 steps in a week, gives me a sense of accomplishment similar to the amount of work I get done on my walks. But I am compulsive about some things and have created an arbitrary goal for myself. But that's just me and it's only for now. More about that in Chapter 14 on Guilt Walking. If walking the dog gives satisfaction, who's to judge? It works for the dog owner. It's a reason to walk and it has nothing to do with the fitness of the dog owner, only the fitness of the dog.

But all this talk about exercise, stretching, and their benefits. That's not why I walk. The exercise is a side benefit that I gladly accept and value, but is not the reason for my walking. I could get exercise any number of places, like the gym, which I don't like much, riding a bicycle, something I haven't done for years, or even running, but I don't think so. I enjoy my walks. On the days when I find it difficult or impossible to walk, I miss it.

I am not alone in walking for something other than exercise. My neighbor John is a prime example. John recently got a new dog. For years, John walked his old dog, Chloe, in the neighborhood. Well, later on, "walking" was an exaggeration. She had gotten so old that her walks involved going from shrub to shrub sniffing. Even though she couldn't even go around the block, John took her out several times a day. Finally, Chloe went to doggie heaven and could sniff as much as she wanted, and John got a new dog, Daisy. He takes her out several times a day, too, but I see him far from home now his dog walking him. His reason is he walks for Daisy.

Do dog owners walk for their dogs? A study mostly from the University of Liverpool, England, and published in the *International Journal of Environmental Research and Public Health*, found that "Dog walking was constructed as 'for the dog,' however, owners represented their dog's needs in a way which aligned with their own. . . . Owners reported deriving positive outcomes from dog walking, most notably, feelings of 'happiness,' but these were 'contingent' on the perception that their dogs were enjoying the experience." They took walking their dogs as a "responsibility," not to themselves but to the dog. Someone named Adam was quoted in the study, "The best way to put it is, see him as yourself and if you get fat you don't like it and he won't like it.

Maybe he'll go on a downer, I don't know, but I'm trying to keep him fit and healthy and treat him like I am myself."

Dog walking does get people off the sofa and onto the sidewalk, though. Another English study from the Norwich Medical Center found that fewer than 50 percent of "older adults" were sufficiently physically active, but that dog walkers were far more active than people without dogs to take "responsibility" for.

The "walk-ecstatic dog" is inspiration for setting foot out the door to take the dog for a walk Just the sight of a leash sends a dog into paroxysms of joy, something that may just brighten the dog owner's day and gets him or her out the door "for the dog." I don't own a dog, even though John tells me I need to get one, but I don't intend to. Dog walking is not on any of my lists for reasons to walk, and besides dogs are a lot of trouble. You can't go anywhere on trips without considerable accommodation for the dog. You have to bathe them regularly, something most dogs would rather not and will let you know in various irritating ways. You have to take them to the vet, what most dogs hate more than baths. You have to feed them with the "right" kind of food. And you have to pick up the poop they deposit willy-nilly on their walks.

Of course, all this discussion about the proper number of steps, stiffness, and dog walking can make someone feel like a failure if he or she doesn't "measure up" to some artificial standard or have a "reason" to go for a walk.

Mostly my walks are to be alone, see new things, see old things in a new way, and old things I never saw before. They are to enjoy my excursions into nature and the city. One day recently I sat in the shade of a tree in the desert listening to the songs of the birds and the hum of civilization, traffic, backup beeps, an airplane overhead. I have time to do that because I don't have to be anywhere or do anything, usually. I divorce myself from things I have to do as much as I can on my walks. That day, I just wanted to sit and soak in the morning. Without stiffness, the walk is ever more pleasant, productive, and satisfying. I feel a walk coming on.

Chapter 8
The Productivity Trap

I tell myself, "well anyway, I enjoyed the walk, but I'll do better next time." But deep down inside my psyche, submerged in my brain, it's growling that I am fooling myself. I haven't been "productive." I've trapped myself. I didn't get two pages of notes, an article worked out so I can sit down and write it when I get back, or didn't think through a problem and a solution that might actually work. I have set up arbitrary requirements for a walk.

This chapter came to me on one of those days when I did come up with "something useful." It exploded in my brain on a walk. Obviously, it had been bubbling up, trapped in a pressure cooker, waiting for a chance to escape and enter my consciousness. The inspiration was that we don't always need to be doing something "useful," "something "productive" is the point of this chapter. But at the time this idea exploded in my brain, I thought what a terrific walk it had been and that I would remember it as one of the best walks ever. I ensnared myself in the productivity trap.

Most of the other chapters in this book deal with the psychic rewards of a walk, the peace it brings, the mindfulness it encourages, the quiet mind it results in. Yet, here I am complaining about not getting two or three pages of notes, an article worked through, a problem solved. Most of the other times, it isn't productivity that makes a walk valuable, even though I do work when I walk and do get things sorted out on a walk. But flipping the switch off from the Zen experience to the "productivity experience," I have come to think is self-defeating, leaving out important rewards a walk can bring. Still, here I am with the dilemma.

What is "productivity"? What is "useful"? What is getting something "done"? It depends whom you ask. Should that be the only reason to go for a walk? For me productivity has to be allowed to find its own way, with the understanding that sometimes trying to force it shuts it off. My mastermind group read the book *The Productivity Project* by Chris Bailey in which the author describes the techniques he has used to make himself more productive. Oh so many gyrations and convolutions he went through. He describes how some things worked and how some things didn't. Even though it is a good book, it poisoned my mind. He constantly forced himself to be productive, but didn't always give his brain the chance to work on things without his forcing it, that is until later. Eventually, he talks about meditating, and it is part of being "productive." That, of course, is one reason to meditate and go for walks. And becoming more productive is one of the primary reasons I walk, but it has chains and padlocks, things I will talk about in a minute.

Chris Bailey got the book written, edited, published, and put on the market, and good for him, That was a huge accomplishment.

We read the book to help us become more productive in our businesses. But still I wonder if Chris Bailey's ideas are everything I need in order to not only be more productive but to get my brain to do what I intend. Is forcing my brain into a crammed tiny space what I need or intend? And is productivity important? And is what I intend influenced by Bailey?

Here's my dilemma and problem: I work when I walk, using walks to get ideas and chapters sorted out. On this particular walk, I got almost four pages of notes in the three miles or so I put one foot in front of the other. At first, I remembered the University of Michigan study I wrote about in Chapter 6 about how walking in nature resets the brain. The study, you may recall, showed that our brains can jettison Directed Attention Fatigue when we escape the places that demand constant attention, such as city streets with traffic, people, and other civilization distractions. Walking in nature, the study showed, enables us to restore our attention. The study only dealt with one aspect, a memory test, but that's the only evidence they had the right to conclude from. Having no such strictures, I can speculate, I can generalize, and I can propose ideas about how resetting my mind can benefit me, making me more productive.

The ideas flowed when I started on the nature part of my walk. It's a half mile to the beginning of nature and a couple of ideas managed to seep out before I got there. But once I got to where the city stopped and nature started, everything spewed out and fed on itself to make what I believe is a valid conclusion about how this brain resetting: this ken, reflective, experience is productive.

On my walk, ideas came unbidden in no particular order or sequence. I wrote them down as I thought of them, and sometimes I could barely get one written down before the next one gushed into my head. I would have almost jumped for joy if I had set out to think something through and get specific ideas. My brain took me in an entirely different direction, though, one where it wanted, or needed, to go. I might have been looking at productivity all wrong, at least consciously.

Here's the problem, if it is one, and maybe the key to unlock the padlock. So far this book has had a bewildering tendency to discuss increasing my productivity through walking—all mixed in with the vision of ken. But as I thought of during my walk, the brain doesn't always do, maybe rarely does, what it's told. Giving it direction means asking the right question. I remember one *Twilight Zone* episode, "The Man in the Bottle," it's Episode 38, if you want to watch it on YouTube, where an antique shop owner kindly bought a magic lamp from a needy old woman, paying too much for it, then dutifully rubbed it. He got four wishes, the first one to prove that the genie was actually capable of granting the wishes. Of course, the lucky shop owner blurted out wishes without thinking through the ramifications of those wishes. It was the ultimate "be careful what you wish for" scenario. Telling the brain what to think about can lead to the same sort of "be careful" even though we are more in control of it than a genie from a bottle would allow us to be.

I have been working on how to tell my brain what to think about. I have asked myself how to make it so specific that it can't go wandering off on side journeys or even on a separate trip that ends up nowhere near the answers I told it to come up with. Instead it has given me "answers" I should have been careful not to have asked for. I have trapped myself in productivity.

This chapter notwithstanding, the key for me is to have an end in mind before I ask my brain to come up with the step-by-step procedure for getting there. And even at that, the notes I came up with on my walk had no particular organization but were just confused stream of consciousness. That's a challenge because I am a global learner, so I must have the "big picture" before I can formulate the steps or even understand the steps. I had all the steps, but no particular end in mind. Many other people learn best sequentially, step-by-step, and that works for them. But when I see or hear a step-by-step method or procedure and I have no idea of where it is going to end up, mostly what I think is "so what." Thus, if I begin with a description of a point a chapter of this book will make, I am more likely to come up with the steps necessary to get there. But if I just start with telling my brain to for example "come up with ideas about a chapter on competitive walking," it goes off on its own direction, or directions, and usually ending up with not much of anything, useful or useless. In the case of this chapter, my brain was off on its own direction but gave me enough material to create an organization that mostly works, albeit with considerable editing and revision.

Here's my trap. My definition or idea of productivity and the word "done" need revision. I get caught up in numbers, goals, and results, and whether I have met the numbers, accomplished the goals, and gotten the results I wanted. As I have walked more and more, as I have become more and more fit by working with a trainer, as I have admired how well I am doing, I became results oriented rather than satisfaction oriented, with results that made no real difference. The results took on a life of their own.

If I don't meet a number, maybe I don't need to work harder, to force myself but rather need to readjust reasons for walking. I know all the techniques for generating ideas and promoting progress such as using mindstorming that I wrote about in Chapter 5. The numbers, the "progress," become more important, and the reason I have for walking becomes overshadowed by averages and standard deviations, p- and t-values, and deciding if I have walked "enough." Then, when I do better than average, I can pat myself on the back and tell myself, "good work."

When I think about productivity, I often concern myself with keeping track of things because then I know I have been "productive." My productivity need not include how many words or pages I wrote or ideas I got. As a reflective learner, before I can understand anything well enough to discuss it and write about it, I need to think it through. So even though I may not be pounding on a keyboard, or pathetically staring at a blank screen, I am working. Then when I put together what I have been thinking about, making notes about, and organizing on a yellow pad, I know how to accomplish what I need to accomplish and it flows out like magic (well, the magic's devoutly to be wished). That even includes the disorganized, random ideas I got when this chapter exploded into my consciousness.

Thus, productive means something different to me than it might to someone else and used to mean to me. I do get things done, sometimes in fits and starts, and sometimes in long periods of churning out what I have allowed my brain to cogitate on, to work on, to formulate because I eventually asked it the right question, properly phrased, or it somehow, without intervention from me, figured out on its own what I needed to do.

Productive doesn't always mean "getting things done," though. Leo Baubata wrote thoughts that expressed exactly why I walk and the pleasure it gives me on mnmlist.com/joy-of-walking.

Today I set out from my house and walked. And walked.

I didn't have a specific destination in mind, but wanted to walk a bit before finding a quiet place to write. So I walked, out of the town where I live and along the tropical, white-sand coastline, to the next town over. . .

As others were productive and got tasks done, I walked and got nothing done, and cleared my head.

As others had the comfort of shelter and air-conditioning, I walked and worked up a light sweat and was buffeted by the wind.

As a white gull floated serenely above a calm bay, I walked, and watched, and loved it.

I walked for an hour, then wrote and read, and then walked for another hour to get back home, tired but happy.

I can't walk this much every day, but I walk as much as I can, because you need nothing to walk, you spend nothing, you consume nothing, you emit nothing.

And yet you have everything.

If you liked this post, feel free to use it. Leo posted, "No permission is needed to copy, distribute, or modify the content of this site. Credit is appreciated but not required."

Here's the flip side. There's no telling what you'll get when you let the genie out of the lamp. That's neither good nor bad, just what you make it. What you get may be exactly what you need when you let the brain out of its productivity trap. Could it be that productivity is also peace of mind or an empty brain?

Is productivity in terms of getting things done important? Of course, it is, but the definition is far from straightforward. I need to get work done, to accomplish what I want to accomplish. But I can get caught in the trap of trying to be "productive." That means I make schedules, keep track of "progress" or accomplishment, and in the process create arbitrary rules for myself that often are unnecessary. Yes, rules and goals usually work to accomplish things, but what might I miss by pounding myself into the productivity trap square hole for my round head, or round hole with my square head?

The vision experience of ken requires being mindfully in the present moment, in this case to walk to enjoy the moment, to contemplate the world, to reset the brain. It works better reset, after all. I need to differentiate between the seemingly urgent, the arbitrary rules I create, and the important. Some things are both urgent and important, but usually not. I want to escape the productivity trap and free myself to do the important in a way that results in quality work, work that deserves to last. In the words of that famous philosopher Mick Jagger, "You can't always get what you want/ But if you try sometimes, you just might find/ You get what you need."

I feel a walk coming on.

Chapter 9
Joyful Walking

We called her Joyless, at least Jason and I did. Joy, her real name, was the paymaster where I worked, and she had never been known to even hint at a smile. You'd think that she would have derived at least some joy or pleasure out of the outstanding job she did getting 1200-plus people paid accurately every week, and maybe she did, but apparently that wasn't cause for even an inkling of demonstrated pleasure, much less joy. My wife suggested that she had personal problems she didn't share. Regardless, she was still Joyless.

I'm not sure what joy is, though. There's pleasure, and I know what that is. People get pleasure out of all kinds of activities and events. Richard Wagner suggested, "Joy is not in things; it is in us." I get pleasure out of walking most days. Others get pleasure out of a job well done, a hobby, a study, and many other things. I know a man who gets pleasure out of the five classic cars he owns and drives in rotation. A carpenter gets pleasure out of doing craftsman-like work. A plumber gets pleasure out of making a permanent repair to a plumbing problem or even plumbing an entire house the most efficacious way. An artist gets pleasure out of creating a piece that communicates exactly what she had in mind. A writer gets pleasure out of a piece of writing that creates a feeling of pride in his craft. That's happened to me a couple of times. Then, imagine Thomas Edison's pleasure, when on what turned out to be the successful trial of the light bulb when it stayed lit 13-and-a-half hours. He might even have experienced joy then.

What I do know is that joy spreads out and infects everything around it. Many others are like me and delight in being around joyful people. These folks light up a room, or any area, even out in nature where they are inspired by the experience and radiate joy. Energy radiates from them, and it improves everyone's mood. Of course, negative energy radiates, too, and unless your mood is also negative and you want to compete with that person about who is most cynical and unhappy, you get out of their way as quickly as possible.

I am disturbed by those who denigrate joy or pleasure in everyday activities or occupations. Henry David Thoreau is an especially self-righteous and irritating example. He ranted in his essay "Walking," "You may safely say, A penny for your thoughts, or a thousand pounds. When sometimes I am reminded that the mechanics and shopkeepers stay in their shops not only all the forenoon, but all the afternoon too, sitting with crossed legs, so many of them—as if the legs were made to sit upon, and not to stand or walk upon—I think that they deserve some credit for not having all committed suicide long ago."

Okay, so you find pleasure in walking, Henry. So do I. "Mechanics and shopkeepers" may find joy in their jobs. People can find joy in anything they do; it is up to each person to find out what gives him or her joy however described.

But this chapter is about joyful walking, not about the joy people may find in other things. I just had to disabuse anyone of the notion that I thought walking was the only avenue to joy.

> "Sometimes you never know the value of a moment until it becomes a memory."—*Zig Ziglar*

Remember the quote from Leo Baubata in Chapter 8? I particularly like how he ended his essay.

> I can't walk this much every day, but I walk as much as I can, because you need nothing to walk, you spend nothing, you consume nothing, you emit nothing.

> And yet you have everything.

Was Leo joyful? I can't say if he would have described that particular walking experience as joy, but he seems to have thoroughly enjoyed it. I am trying to find a way to remember wonderful, joy-filled walks I have taken. I distinctly remember walks that were neither wonderful nor joyful, such as those where I managed to get injured. But I have trouble remembering joy or even describing what joy is.

Just what is joy? It is an emotion where we may remember how happy we were. Mindbodygreen.com describes it as "When we feel joy, we feel great about ourselves. We feel confident, powerful, capable, lovable and fulfilled." They have pills for that. Adjectives mean something only to the person who uses them, and maybe not even then—just words. But of course, joy is subjective. I don't know if I am even qualified to talk about joy because I am not sure how to describe it so even I can say to myself, "I am joyful now."

My aim is to find techniques for enabling joy in my walks. That's one reason I decided to write about walking and particularly the vision experience of ken walking. We looked at mindful walking in that chapter with techniques for clearing the mind, not becoming joyful. I clear my mind so I can work on what I believe is important, or just enjoy the day, or both. Mindbodygreen.com suggests another idea, "Do an uplifting and enjoyable activity that's not goal-oriented, but just plain fun." Well, maybe, but is that the only way?

Cloud nine, walking on air, grin from ear to ear, music to your ears, best day ever, pumped, stoked, I can't believe it!, happy as a flea in a doghouse, over the moon, in seventh heaven, thrilled to bits, tickled pink, on top of the world all provide visuals and to me indicate joy. Maybe these are the best ways to describe it.

My youngest brother, David, got what the family called Christmas Eveitis. He was so excited about Christmas that he got physically ill every Christmas Eve until he was probably 10 years old. He anticipated the joy he would experience as he opened presents Christmas morning. It was a joke with the family but real joy to him every year. Even as an adult, he enjoyed Christmas so much because of the joy he counted on experiencing from the gifts he would receive. Anticipation of an event that is sure to put you on cloud nine, make you grin from ear to ear, put you over the moon, or make you thrilled to bits makes joy. Now, how to experience it?

The question arises, do we have to clear our minds before we can experience joy, or can joy come after building anticipation and excitement about an event? I don't know, and I don't suppose it matters.

I can summon up ideas I have heard and read about experiencing joy. Mostly I have forgotten about them because I am busy regurgitating all that unpleasant stuff. One thing that comes up over and over is gratitude. Does gratitude automatically create joy? Most likely not. Gratitude works because it uses a different part of the brain that has no use for negativity, or so say those who should know. Negativity must be banished, at least temporarily, if we are to experience joy, but its absence doesn't necessarily mean we are joyful.

My granddaughter, Victoria, who is in her early 20s, is the most grateful person I know. Every morning, she has told me, first thing she thinks of all the things she is grateful for. She has a list, and she goes over it. As a result, she is joyful and a pleasure to be around. I envy her. Success has resulted from her gratitude and joy. She seems to be successful at everything she does and tries and relishes every fantastic adventure she experiences.

Why don't I make such a list? Then, on my walks when my thoughts revert to the unpleasant, to the dredging up of events that have negatively affected my life, to amplifying them infinitely past any possible importance, I can just think about the many things I am grateful for. But that is not so easy considering my lifelong practice, petulance, and predilection.

How do I turn on gratitude? The first thing is to think of things I am grateful for. That's the hard part, but I made a list. I have plenty to be grateful for, and I will think more about those things. My grumble usually takes over, but maybe gratitude will win out. It's mostly my upbringing because I was raised in a household that gloried in the negative. They could turn a positive into something to worry about in three or four words, "yeah, but," "what if." Amazing how they could do that. But I don't want to be like that.

We have looked at tricks for resetting the brain in previous chapters, such as walking in nature and even walking backwards, maybe in nature, walking mindfully. But there's more.

One thing I have seen numerous times is the suggestion to smile. That is supposed to communicate to the brain that we are happy. I know it works most of the time, but nothing, of course, works all the time.

Then there is breathing. If we take several slow, deep breaths, that is supposed to generate Alpha waves (relaxing) and abate Beta waves (stress). I tried, sitting here in front of the computer to both smile and breathe, and, in spite of the fact that I wasn't rummaging into my past for negatives, it may have relaxed me. We looked at how breathing can encourage mindful meditation in Chapter 6 along with counting steps. It clears the head and enables us to put more pleasantness in our thoughts.

Another way is a playlist of songs that make me happy. I thought of that on occasion, but hadn't followed through on it until now. I created a playlist, a work in progress, in which every song makes me smile or at least feel happy. I don't want to listen to music when I walk, but have no problem at all with it when sitting and working. One of my favorites is Vivaldi's Flute Concertos that always makes me at least smile. Others are "Mr. Blue Sky" by

Electric Light Orchestra, "I Just Called to Say I Love You" by Stevie Wonder, and "Betcha Bygolly, Wow" by The Stylistics.

I know there are other ways to encourage joy, and I will work on them, too. But this book is about walking and this chapter about joyful walking, so that's what I am coming back to.

If I try, I can remember some joyful walks I have taken. Those give me happiness looking back on as much as they did when I took them. There were the walks I mentioned in Chapter 1 in Forest Park in Portland with my wife, children, and dog Oliver. There was the walk my wife and I took in the Redwoods a few years ago. There were the walks my wife and I took in Forest Park in Portland when we decided to explore all the trails, years after our children were grown and out of the nest. One particular walk recently I remember was when I sat awhile in the shade of a tree and drank in nature. No, I don't remember the date, but it's in my notebook where I could look it up if I wanted, but forever written in my memory.

Then there was the walk I began at 5:30 on a Sunday morning. Not another soul was out and the birds were in full song. I had the world to myself. Finally, one man showed up in the street coming toward me walking his dog, but I had turned off onto another street by then. I got to the desert to continue my walk and the temperature dropped 15 degrees. It felt cold. My thermometer at home said it was 67 degrees when I started, on its way to 105 degrees later. It was a joy-filled walk, completely undiluted by the martini the night before.

Getting joy out of walking, and joy more often is my plan, not just during the walk, but in my memory. How do I go about that? That, of course, is the exploration and adventure. I don't believe we can go out and make joy happen; we just have to permit it to happen, encourage it, and delight in it when it does. I wish there were a magic formula, or a magic lamp that I could rub, that would generate a joyful walk every time I set foot out the front door for my daily adventure, but I have yet to find it in spite of my extensive explorations. Even without "joy," walks are worthwhile more often than not. Since I work when I walk, when I think through an article or chapter, get ideas for a piece of writing, figure out the solution to a problem, the walk is satisfying and enjoyable, and maybe even brimming with joy since I sorted out what I needed and wanted to write. And, so, I may be joyful about the results of my walk, even if it isn't "an intense and especially ecstatic or exultant happiness." My wife suggests, I am "tightly wound." Maybe it's time to at least loosen the tension. I do want to avoid my own perception that I am joyless.

Above all, do not lose your desire to walk: every day I walk myself into a state of well-being and walk away from every illness; I have walked myself into my best thoughts and I know of no thought so burdensome that one cannot walk away from it.— *Søren Kierkegaard*

I feel a walk coming on, and I know it will be both a productive and, as I wish, a joyful one.

Chapter 10
"See If I Can" Walking

Remarkable

Deserving notice or comment; worthy of remark or attention.
Hence: striking, unusual, singular. (OED)

Almost 650 people climbed Mt. Everest in 2017, and I would guess about all of them just hoped to get to the summit with no thought of being fastest, oldest, youngest, or anything else "-est." The average time for completing the Iron Man Triathlon is about 14 hours 20 minutes with the world record 7:39:25. Obviously the vast majority of participants have no hope or intention of winning or setting a record. Sara Palacios swam the English Channel in 2018 in a time of 12 hours 58 minutes, but never thought of setting the world record for the swim, which is for a one-way swim 6 hours 55 minutes. I ran four marathons, albeit decades ago, with not even a glimmer of an idea of winning since I couldn't run even one four-minute forty-one second mile much less 26 in a row, about what would be required to equal a world record.

They and I do those things not to win but to see if we can. Think of it as contests with ourselves. As the Ironman official website sums up the reason, "Ironman is about persevering, enduring and being a part of something larger than ourselves." To some people, it is an obsession. To them, it is never being satisfied with "good." Rather it is doing something to be proud of. And to them, it is wanting to "see if they can" and then beaming with pride for their accomplishments, for milestones, for a revelation of "yeah, I did it!" As a result, they do remarkable things, (except me because I don't think of what I do or did as "remarkable").

One remarkable exception to the lack of a record-setting goal was by my friend George Meegan who was the first, and I believe only, person to walk the entire length of the Western Hemisphere. As he wrote in his book *The Longest Walk*, "I had discovered that what I truly longed for were the exotic lands that always beckoned beyond the horizon. In my country's tradition of grand adventure, I yearned to make my own effort, perhaps even my own mark." He had to see if he could. And he did see if he could, and completed the remarkable journey.

For many people who achieve "great" things, it is at least partially to impress others, maybe to become famous. Possibly they do it to get sponsorship for their activity, such as walking across the country or sailing around the world. They do something they have wanted to do for many days, months or even years and can't wait to let people know what they did. That's fine for them, but "great" things need not be anything that we share with other people. They can be things we do for ourselves, things we consider great. That's almost always the way I aim to approach not just my walks but all my goals.

We all know the goal thermometers. You know the posters showing how close an organization is to accomplishing its goal of raising whatever amount of money. We see the red gauge climb toward success. It doesn't happen all at once. Neither does accomplishing personal goals.

I have found that "seeing if I can" may be the most memorable and rewarding approach to walking and feeding motivation. Obviously, it can't be done all at once. It works best incrementally, a step at a time or walk at a time. Like any goal setting worth spending much effort on, satisfaction comes with achieving intermediate goals each step of the way. Seeing if I can may involve a long-term goal such as the ultimate climbing of Mt. Everest (no, I have not even a scintilla of a brain cell considering that), but there's no way anyone would think of climbing Mt. Everest next week after never having climbed more than a half-mile steep hill or contemplate swimming the English Channel after swimming 10 laps in the pool. The best part is that even incremental goals can be just as satisfying.

Few, if any, of my walks are or even aim at being remarkable, but occasionally one of them is, sometimes even intentionally. Why would a walk sometimes be remarkable? I walk places, usually not to do anything special, but simply to enjoy the walk, soak in nature and/or to get work done. But other times, I get the bizarre notion to push myself.

I am not competitive, so I don't try, want to, or care if I beat anyone else, walk faster than anyone else, walk farther than anyone else. In fact, if I see someone walking ahead of me, I won't even try to catch up and pass. I might even slow down or change my route so I don't catch up. But I can be so proud if I outdo myself, not someone else, or I accomplish a "let's see if I can" walk. Let's see if I can walk all the way to . . . . Let's see if I can climb those hills. Let's see if I can walk to the shopping center and not have to rest up for two hours after I come back. Let's see if I can walk 10 miles and still be able to get out of bed, and even walk the next day. Let's see if I can do anything out of the ordinary, at least my ordinary, be proud of myself, and enjoy the walk. Let's see if I can do something that is remarkable *for me.*

Especially important is to be true to my own abilities since I am on the slippery side of life. I don't recover in an hour or so, or even a day or so if I push too hard. But I can push a little any given day and build up to what had been way too hard. I have noticed that over the last couple of years, I can walk more now than I had thought possible even a year before and still go out and relish my walk the next day.

The best part is that no one has to or needs to know. I may have goals, even written goals, but I wouldn't dream of sharing them with anyone whom I don't trust implicitly, and not even those people most of the time. They are my accomplishments for my own satisfaction, not to compare with anyone else. In fact, I rarely share any of my accomplishments just because they are mine and mine only. One of my biggest irritations is people who want to one-up someone else. "Oh, that's nothing. . . " I don't want anyone else's approval or praise even though I will praise another person's accomplishment. And I will never "one-up" another person. Another person's accomplishments are his or hers alone and worthy of congratulations, not comparison, unless maybe, that person is trying to beat a record or another remarkable performance. I just say "good job" and "congratulations," and may ask him or her how it all came about. "Seeing if I can" has nothing to do with what anyone else does. There doesn't have to be a winner except oneself.

Walking for me isn't about anyone else. It's about what I want to get out of it. I make a point of not boring people with something I have accomplished even if they ask. My own satisfaction is enough.

My "see if I cans" may not even be a physical accomplishment. I may see if I can get some fantastic new ideas. I may see if I can calm my mind. I may see if I can walk mindfully for 10 minutes. I may see if I can see 10 things that I have never seen before on my walk. I may see if I can get some new insight into a situation, idea, or thought.

Are these non-physical "see if I cans" appropriate? I don't see why not. I ask, is "seeing if I can" exclusive to physical activity? But nobody determines my walk's goals except me, the person who's going for a walk. If I want to make that morning's goal seeing 10 things I have never seen before, how could that be anything but right? After all, I walk for my reasons and no one else's.

I am going to try one of the non-physical ideas for seeing, ken, if I can.

One recent morning's walk I tried to see if I could go the entire walk mindfully. Once I remembered I was going to do that, and that took a couple of blocks, I started counting steps. I did well until I got to a place where I had to pay full attention to where I stepped, but after I finished that part, I started again. I did relatively well but then ideas began to flood into my brain. I got one of the best ideas I have gotten for several months, a subtitle for this book. It's on the cover, "An exploration of the many adventures of a walk." I played with it some more and thought of a variety of slightly different phrases, but that one was the best of the lot. But I never did get back to my mindfulness on that walk. Even so, as I have discovered, mindfully walking has worked wonders for my creativity.

I tried again to walk mindfully the other day and got through the entire walk counting steps. Trouble was, I never got any new ideas or thoughts. I accomplished my goal, but the upshot of the goal wasn't anything but the step counting. And that brings me to the point of setting goals for a walk. What is my reason for the goal? If the accomplishment itself is the reason, that works. But in my case, the accomplishment is so I can accomplish an additional goal. That's where I have to be careful to ask the right questions, to try for the precise end.

Remember the Twilight Zone episode I mentioned in Chapter 8 about "The Productivity Trap"? Counting steps the entire walk wasn't the goal of the walk. The idea of counting steps is to be mindful and think of new ideas and unique ways to express an idea, not just the activity itself. That's where I need to be careful. My goal wasn't to walk mindfully but to count steps, and that didn't lead anywhere but was a means to an end. Or was it?

A walk is more than just a walk, if you want it to be. It is an experience, an exploration, an expectation of a pleasant memory, even if that doesn't always happen. It is those things if I decide it will be. When a walk become an obligation, it lessens its possibility of delight, joy, and seeing if I can.

That brings up the question of how to set a goal for a walk that is both what I want to accomplish and what I can call a benefit to me. The walk where it devolved into thinking up the subtitle for this book was a benefit. But I need to carefully think up things I want to accomplish on a walk that will end up as a benefit so the experience and exploration live up to the expectation.

I feel a walk coming on and expect it to be rewarding and memorable.

Chapter 11
Social Walking

These were no ordinary walks. They were memorable and special, walks I celebrate, walks I remember and treasure. These are walks that delight my memory, some individually, some as part of several walks of the same group of walks. These are walks I fondly think back on, sometimes during my "ordinary" walks. Nothing is "ordinary" about these etch my memory with gratitude. These are walks I took with others.

Virtually all of these walks were with family. I wrote about the walks in Forest Park in Chapter 1 both with my entire family and later with my wife. Those walks' memories I treasure. There were also the walks I took with my children and grandchildren when they visited one Christmas. We walked a couple of my favorite routes, routes where you rarely see other walkers and nature abounds so they could all enjoy the peace of walking in nature.

My wife's and my walk in the Redwoods resulted in some of our greatest joy. We walked the two-point-four-mile Drury-Chaney Loop on the Avenue of the Giants through the Redwoods on a vacation a couple of years ago. What an experience! Yes, there were a few other people there, but they weren't there to be sociable, just as we weren't. So it was just my wife and me reveling in the towering trees that mostly block out the sunlight but show glimpses of the sky trying its best to peek through the treetops. The scrumptious aroma of the forest, the fallen trees and snags, some of which were one-story high with paths of their own on top, and the side paths that went places just as interesting as the main path, or maybe more so, or went nowhere in particular, and of course the trees are what are forever etched in memory. Time stood still as we relished our excursion through the forest.

Then there was the walk my wife and I took when we visited our daughter and her husband in Oakland. I remember the stairs. The prodigious flight of stairs starts at the east side of Oak Glen Park on Richmond Blvd. and climbs a bazillion steps to Kempton Ave. above. I had to climb it. After all, no way could I let my daughter and son-in-law think I was a wimp. There was nothing special about Kempton Ave., just houses, albeit expensive houses even by Oakland's obscene housing price standards, so we came back down. But the climb was rewarding and, obviously, memorable.

Oak Glen Park is itself a pleasant place to walk, what with the creek, the paths and the bridges over the creek. Apparently, it wasn't always so pleasant. The park's history is inherently more interesting than the stairs or the park itself. The story has it that the entire area was once owned by A.J. Pope who raced and trained his horses in Oak Glen Park with the horses drinking out of Glen Echo Creek, which runs through the park. Glen Echo Creek was created in 1912 (there's lots of water running under Oakland) but not cared for with any noticeable diligence by the city of Oakland. In 1955, some 200 people signed a petition declaring that the creek was "a public health hazard, a grave danger to our children and a public nuisance" and demanded the creek be filled. The city of Oakland responded by turning the creek and the lands either side of it over to the state of California thus relieving the city of the responsibility for keeping the mosquitos at bay, preventing garbage dumping, and diverting responsibility for preventing child molestation to state government.

I can understand people who like to walk with others. They enjoy being with other people. They may need the obligation of a scheduled walk to prompt them to put walking shoes on their feet and their feet out the door. Nothing wrong with that, so don't think that I am implying there is. It's simply not something I want to do, what with my asocial proclivities and all.

Social walking opportunities abound. One organized social walk program combines social walking and medical care, Walk With a Doc. Their website says, "By creating a safe environment to experience health education and inspiration. Oh, and you'll get your steps in for the day too!" One local website says, "While you walk at your own pace, you'll have the opportunity to have questions answered by local physicians. At each walk you'll receive FREE heart-healthy snack, wonderful conversations and walking (with a Doc)! And new participants will receive a free t-shirt!" Gee, free food and t-shirt, what else could you want? Sign me up! The Walk With a Doc website also lists 100 reasons to walk. I looked at them and each has something to do with health ranging from cholesterol fixes to number 100 "The Surgeon General calls us to Step it Up." It's as if walking is a prescription. But what else can you expect out of a program organized by doctors?

Here in Tucson in the summer, the outdoor walks are on hiatus since it's likely to be more than 90 degrees outside by the time the walk is finished even if they start at 6 AM. So they walk at a mall. I don't fancy walking at a mall, but I had to find out for myself about walking with a doc, so I went to the first monthly outdoor event after the weather cooled. I wondered what the t-shirt would look like and the "healthy snack" would be, but I never found out since neither appeared. Eight people did appear for the walk, though. Before we started the walk, the doctor in charge of that walk, who will not be named, an admitted vegetarian, talked about 20 minutes about nutrition, mostly with information that I thought was common knowledge but with a couple of interesting takes. One thing she mentioned was that eating French Fries is as bad as smoking. Wow! So eat some fries and it's like smoking a pack of cigarettes? Then there were the statements that eating steak is "questionable," our diets should consist of 20 percent protein, 30 percent fat, and 50 percent carbohydrates, and that eating toast is okay as long as it's not brown. Isn't that the definition of toast, browned bread? I think I'll stick to my own dietary regimen.

The walk began and the doctor talked to different people during the walk that went along a well-traveled walking and bike path. I have never liked walking on that path because the bicycles often go by at 30 miles per hour or so. I spoke to several of the participants about why they came to this walk and mostly it was for the social aspect rather than the draw of talking to a doctor. One woman walks regularly and keeps at it by using a walking game on her phone. I will look at some of those games in the chapter on exercise.

Numerous other opportunities exist for social walking, though. Meetup groups and walking clubs are plentiful and are said to encourage walking. Lifehacker.com writes "A meta study from the *British Journal of Sports Medicine,* a summation of 42 individual studies involving 1,843 participants, showed that overall, people who walked small amounts received a wide range of mental and physical benefits. Moreover, people who joined walking groups stuck with their walking routines more than people who didn't."

Then there are the dog walkers. There's a website for dog walking social groups. They promise, "These groups are a terrific opportunity for any dog, reactive or not, to socialize with canine pals. Contrary to popular beliefs, off leash play isn't the only game in town when it comes to socialization. Side by side walks on leash and training classes are social activities for your dog too!" You may remember dog walking as a reason for exercise in Chapter 7, "Seniors' Walking."

The Mayo Clinic has the most enticing come on for social walking, "Walking group: Banish boredom, boost motivation. Starting a walking group requires little effort and provides big rewards. Simply spread the word and get organized. Soon you'll be walking toward better health." They add "You already know the health benefits of walking. Here's what else you get when you walk with others:

- Accountability
- Motivation
- Safety
- Socialization"

They are the medical profession, after all, so they have to push health. At least they start off with banishing boredom and boosting motivation. And they did add accountability and motivation albeit as side benefits. They left off my reasons for walking, though, the insight of ken and diversion experiences, the chance to think things through, the freedom to work. But I am just a little less sociable than many other people.

I would walk even if there were no health benefit. And when you get down to it, health benefits are not the cure-all that health sites make walking out to be. We'll get into that in the exercise chapter. No, it doesn't hurt—usually. And usually it does make you feel better and sometimes more energized, as long as you don't walk too far, something I have a tendency to do and might have done more times than I can count. Then it hurts, but not too much.

The trouble is, for me and I imagine most other people, as I mentioned before, when something becomes an obligation, something we are expected to do, resentment eventually creeps in and we stop looking forward to it and instead dread it. The end result is stopping altogether, thinking of reasons not to do it, rationalizing that you have more important things to do, that walking is taking "too much time." Even though those social walks I mentioned varied from memorable to treasured, I would not want to take walks with family or another person every day. What makes those walks I took with others special is that they didn't happen every day, every week, or even once a month. They were one-off events. If they happened with regularity, they would lose their allure and attraction ending up as nothing to look forward to or back on. In fact, most likely they would end up feeling like an obligation. Obligations get old, tired, and dreaded before long.

So I walk alone, mostly. Walking alone lets me set my own schedule, pace and route. Walking with others requires coordination and planning and accommodating the pace and physical condition of others. It's wonderful every so often but not if it is expected or required.

On my "ordinary" walks, I often have a specific purpose in mind. They are walks I take just about every day and give me a chance to work and maybe, sometimes get my head straight. Well, I work at getting it straight, anyway. On my "ordinary" walks, I walk alone. They give me the opportunity to think through ideas, to work out articles, to enjoy the world around me, to be "lonely as a cloud," minus the daffodils per Wordsworth. One walk, though, I did see fields of blooming brittle bush, a golden carpeted hillside. I took a picture of that, but nothing else about that walk stands out.

I work best alone. Mostly it's because I am not particularly sociable, and walking with other people would require me to be sociable. I value my time alone. Nothing new there. I recently saw my report card from second grade (my mother had kept it) where the teacher wrote that I was not getting along on the playground, not being sociable enough. Just think, an entire life of nonsocial existence. That was one of the years I walked home from school in Chula Vista, California, alone with myself and my thoughts, whatever those might have been.

Walking does take time, but not "too much," and I value the time I walk. My reasons for walking have nothing to do with any obligation except to myself, so I don't resent the time it takes. Those reasons have to do with enjoyment and peace and quiet and the ability to contemplate, ruminate, cogitate, find joy, see if I can, explore, and write. If I were doing it solely for exercise or to socialize, I know that within about three weeks, I would have found a hundred reasons not to. But instead, after decades of walking, I still almost without fail look forward to my daily jaunts, seeing what I can see, coming up with creative ideas, and marveling at the world.

I feel a walk coming on.

Chapter 12
Competitive Walking

The English aristocracy created a new gambling game around 1600. They bet on their footmen. Footmen already accompanied them when they traveled. Away from the manor house, those duties involved first, walking and running alongside a nobleman's carriage to ensure that the coach didn't overturn by hitting ditches and tree roots, and second, carrying messages and documents and running ahead of the family coach to arrange for food and lodging at inns or advising the staff at the aristocrat's country house that the boss was on his way. When I think about it, though, I can't imagine someone holding up a carriage about to tip over from a rut or tree root.

Mundane purpose was not enough. After all, we have these big, strong boys who are no doubt superior to Lord Jones's or Lord Smith's. Why not prove it and compete with other aristocrats for title (and money) of whose footman is fastest? The game involved betting large sums of money on matches between footmen for speed and stamina. Apparently the rules were few or winked at. The expression "fair heel and toe" came into play sometimes, but as is reported in the book *The Sport of Racewalking*, footmen were "allowed to trot, as necessary, to ward off cramp." So apparently just about anything was acceptable.

In their book *Racewalking*, William Finley and Marion Weinstein report "betting reached such a height that spectators stood along the highway eagerly placing their wagers as the contestants passed." Thus was born the sport of "pedestrianism."

Naturally, the qualification for employment as a footman expanded some to include walking pace and ability to walk long distances. Taller, longer-legged footmen thus earned higher pay. And lest they collapse from hunger, footmen carried a long cane with a mixture of eggs and white wine. And to ensure they received proper restoration at the end of the race, they were refreshed with champagne, the preferred drink. Consider also that they ran, or trotted, in full footman's livery, made of two or more layers of sturdy, but heavy, wool and often adorned with intricately stitched brocade (heavier yet), that displayed their employers' identity. For the vast majority of the year in England, overheating was most likely not a problem, but on some of the warmer summer days, well. . .

As reported in 1913 in *A Handy Book of Curious Information: Comprising Strange Happenings in the World* by William Shepard Walsh, "One of the last recorded contests was in 1770 between a famous running footman and the Duke of Marlborough, the latter wagering that in his phaeton and four (a four-wheeled, light-weight, open carriage) he would beat the footman in a race from Windsor to London. His Grace won by a very small margin. The poor footman, worn out by his exertions and much chagrined by his defeat, died "of over fatigue," it was said. As recently as 1851, still a long time ago, two running footmen preceded the sheriff and judges and the carriage of the High Sheriff of Northumberland on its way to meet the judges of assize. Two pages, footmen, were "on foot holding on to the door handles of the carriage and running beside it."

Not everyone could have that most enviable job as a footman, though. Thus was born individual accomplishments that created an immensely popular spectator sport and ensured that some stamina-filled men could become nearly as rich as an aristocrat.

Foster Powell, born in 1734, was the first to become a national English "hero," if you will. He was not at the top of the list of people we would think of as heroic. At age 26, he moved from York to London where his first job in London was as a clerk. His coworkers described him as "grave and sedate," in fact even making fun of him as a "milksop and muff." The OED explains that a muff in this context anyway is "A foolish, stupid, feeble, or incompetent person; spec. one who is clumsy or awkward in some sport or manual skill." That all changed when he announced that on Sunday he planned to walk to Windsor and back, about 26 miles each way. "Yeah, right," they said, or however they would have said it then. Irritated, he challenged any of them to walk with him. Two of his co-workers were foolish enough to agree. One lasted only 10 miles and the other a creditable 20 miles, but still had to quit, while Powell finished with energy to spare.

His "heroism" increased from there. Sometimes he raced against other walkers and lost only three times. He did a 40-mile race against one Mr. Richard West, betting 40 guineas, and lost by 100 paces, so the report goes. Mr. West, though, in spite of winning was done in by his exertions and almost died, being taken ill the next day and remaining incapacitated for several months. Powell, though, was fine and ready to go on another walk.

In 1773 on a bet of 1000 guineas (£122,300, $160,000, in today's money), he walked from London to York and back, covering 404 miles in five days, 18 hours, about 72 miles a day. Word got out, and by the time he reached Highgate, north of London, 5,000 people on horseback and in carriages met him and cheered him on into London, about 12 miles. Carl Moritz, the German minister I wrote about in Chapter 2, who walked across England in 1782, might have fared better if he had dressed in footman's livery or was competing as a centurion.

That wasn't a one-off for Powell, either. He did it several times. Even 15 years after his first effort, he walked from London to York and back in five days, 19 hours, 15 minutes. He was only 42 years old, so he was just getting into his prime. Still, in 1790 at the age of 54, he took a bet of 20 to 13 guineas that he could do it again in the same five days, 18 hours he had accomplished it in 1773. With an hour and 15 minutes to spare, he arrived at the finish line and won the bet. He wasn't done. He offered to walk 100 miles the next day for even more money, but no one took him up on it. Powell's fame made him the original centurion. To qualify for that title, someone had to walk 100 miles in 24 hours, something Powell did for the first time in 1777 walking from London Bridge to Canterbury and back, 112 miles, in 24 hours. In 1786, he walked 50 miles out and 50 miles back on the Bath Road in 23 ¼ hours.

What finally did him in was his final walk at age 58 in 1793, when he decided to do the walk from London to York and back faster than he had in 1773. He beat his 1773 time by four hours but the exertion killed him. He died on April 22, 1793 in poverty in spite of the money he had earned or won for his walking exploits.

Another of the most famous "pedestrians" was Captain Barclay (Robert Barclay Allardyce) who became famous for both his speed and endurance. Even when he became an old man, he walked from Thetford to London one day (about 81 miles) and back the next. What made him most remarkable, though, was his walking one mile in each of 1,000 consecutive hours on Newmarket Heath in 1809 for 1,000 guineas.

Barclay was apparently able to accomplish those feats because of the way he walked. Walter Thom in 1813 described "His style of walking is to bend forward the body, and to throw its weight on the knees. His step is short, and his feet are raised only a few inches from the ground."

He was a remarkable fellow all around. A Scot, and described as one of the most athletic men of his time, Barclay reportedly could lift a 250-pound man from the floor to a table with one hand and was an expert in the hammer throw and caber toss. The origin of his name also adds to the interest. Barclay's father, Robert Barclay, Sr., married Sarah Ann Allardyce in 1776, and in recognition of his new wife's noble family, took the last name Allardyce (or Allardice) spelling depending on who's asking, I guess.

Captain Barclay made a fortune with his walking prowess and was nicknamed the "Celebrated Pedestrian" because of his long-distance walking ability. Using his walking prowess, he was guilty of a little "gamesmanship" and "sweetening the pot." Once he is said to have bet 1,000 guineas that he could walk 90 miles in 21 hours. He was said to have had a cold and lost the bet. Then he increased the bet to 2,000 guineas and lost again. On the third try when the bet went to 5,000 guineas, he won with an hour to spare.

One day Barclay rose at 5 AM, walked 30 miles while grouse hunting and then walked home, 60 miles, in 11 hours. In 1808 he walked 130 miles spending two nights without sleep. Barclay's "training method" was purging and sweating and the eating of meat, apparently techniques popular in the 19th Century.

Adding to his all-around athleticism, he took an interest in pugilism and trained Tom Cribb, the bare knuckles Champion of the World in 1807.

Barclay died in 1854 of paralysis after he was kicked by a horse, the horse ending up tougher than he was.

By the early 19th Century, pedestrianism became the most popular sport in England, the betting furious. Of course, its popularity moved to America where up to 25,000 people came to watch pedestrians pass by. The popularity grew until shortly before the Civil War then reclaimed its popularity after. In 1867, a 1,136 mile race from Portland, Maine, to Chicago paid the winner $10,000 ($178,000 in today's money)

Even though pedestrianism was generally considered a game for the lower classes, sporting clubs in large cities still sponsored matches. Walking was the norm but apparently trotting and running was okay, too. Then it grew. By the 1850s, newspapers began to report on sports feats with public interest in pedestrianism ballooning. It was the major pre-Civil War sport and victorious pedestrians took home prize money that equaled 40 years pay working in a factory.

Then there was the riot. The mob was upset on March 10, 1879 because the ticket sellers couldn't sell tickets fast enough so spectators could watch the competition for the Astley Belt, a six-day race that went from early Monday to Saturday night. They broke into Gilmore's Garden, an arena between Fourth and Madison Avenues and 26th and 27th Streets in Manhattan (renamed Madison Square Garden May 31, 1879). The crowd was too much for the two policemen trying to keep order and thcy called in reinforcements who rushed over from another part of Gilmore's Garden. The crowd "held its own" for a while, but eventually the police subdued the crowd after the beatings with clubs "on heads and bodies," until they cleared the lobby of the Garden, reported the New York Times.

Matthew Algeo in his book *Pedestrianism: When Watching People Walk Was America's Favorite Spectator Sport* called it "likely the worst episode of civil unrest in New York City since the Civil War draft riots 16 years before." That's quite an assertion considering that at least two New York riots likely were far worse.

One was the Orange riot of July 12, 1871 where Irish Protestants celebrated the victory of the king of England over

James II. They were met by 1500 police and 5,000 National Guard troops, not to mention the pelting with rocks and crockery the demonstrators took from spectators along their parade route. Then the Tompkins Square Riot of January 13, 1874 in the East Village saw the police bashing heads of thousands of the unemployed who were demonstrating against the lack of work. Just those two might qualify as worse episodes of civil unrest than the Gilmore's Garden fracas.

The sport began to fade and America's favorite pastime eventually turned to baseball. But racewalking wasn't finished. The 1904 Olympics included an 800-yard walk as part of what was to become the decathlon. Racewalking became a separate sport for the 1908 Olympics and remains so. For the 2016 Olympics, the winner of the men's 20-kilometer walk was Wang Zhen of China and the winner of the men's 50-kilometer walk was Matej Tóth of Slovakia. Those are the only two men's distances remaining. The winner of the women's 20-kilometer walk, the only racewalk for women, was Liu Hong of China.

Make something into an Olympic event or Olympic Qualifying event, and strict rules rear their heads. Thus, racewalking has rules about how walkers must take their strides. Unlike running, one of a racewalker's feet must be in contact with the ground at all times. More simply, the walker's front foot must be on the ground when his or her rear foot is raised and the front leg must straighten when it touches the ground. Judges are always watching and walkers who "cross the boundary" between walking and running get a yellow paddle, warning of the infraction. If it appears that a walker has "clearly" violated the rules, a judge sends a red card to the chief judge. Three red cards from three different judges (one judge may not issue multiple red cards to one walker), and the chief judge disqualifies the contestant. Within 100 yards of the finish line, either on a track or road, the chief judge may disqualify a contestant if he or she clearly violates the rules regardless of whether he or she has earned any previous red cards. A contestant is considered to have crossed the finish line when his or her torso crosses, not foot.

The Olympics have a couple more racewalking rules, but the above are the major ones and the ones walkers must be most careful with. I tried walking the way a racewalker is supposed to walk. No thanks. Maybe you get used to it, but it was uncomfortable and pretty much ruined the walking experience. Besides, I am neither competing with anyone nor wanting to compete with anyone. Something else I thought of was that following all those rules and form guidelines just might get in the way of seeing if I can, of stopping to look at interesting sites and sights, of stopping and sitting to take in the day, of ruminating. I might once again see if I can walk like a racewalker, but don't see much point in it. The only possible redeeming feature might be if I could treat the race walking stride like counting steps and let my mind flow.

I also tried walking the way Captain Barclay was described as walking, short steps keeping feet close to the ground and leaning forward. That kind of works but doesn't differ all that much from the way I walk now except for the leaning forward part. I continue to take my mother's dictum when I was growing up to "stand up straight." When I walk the Barclay way did, I notice that I might be just a little less tired. It works best on a paved or at least even surface where I don't have to watch every step to keep from tripping on some hazard on a nature trail.

The early walkers, or pedestrians, didn't have strict guidelines. After all, Barclay and Howell walked hundreds of miles most likely without many spectators most of the way. And the interest and amazement was in how far and fast they could walk not with how flawless their form was.

Amateur racewalking continues. Looking up racewalking clubs on the internet, I found several, but it is not the ubiquitous sport that running is and doesn't have the same respect running does. In fact, there are those who make fun of the sport. For example, Bob Costas called it "whispering loudly."

The brochure of the Marin County, California, club offers these reasons for racewalking. "provides aerobic activity that is kind to your knees; engages all your muscles; releases endorphins that lift your mood; may burn as many calories per hour as running but with a lower risk of injury; is an inexpensive and portable sport, you need only shoes; introduces you to great people and new friends."

A club that looks a little more "forgiving" is the Potomac Valley Track Club, which promises it "is a club for elite and developing athletes, and for people who just want to maintain fitness in an easy comfortable forum. Our motto is 'A club for all ages, all paces and all ways.' Come join us, compete, stay in shape, become a working member and supporter of PVTC, the rewards are great."

In my neighborhood, I sometimes see people "walking with purpose," arms cocked and feet moving with speed and determination. One woman in my neighborhood has been walking fast for several years, but she is the exception. It's unusual to see someone walk purposefully for exercise. As I was researching this chapter, I remembered the Nero Wolfe novella, "Not Quite Dead Enough," set during World War II, when Wolfe, called into the service of his country decides he must thin down and does so by "walking fast." As is the case with most people who walk fast to lose weight and for exercise, Wolfe's notion wore itself out in short order. By far most walkers are simply getting their feet out the door and enjoying the outdoors, and sometimes saying hello to neighbors. That appeals to me more than any alternative except walking alone with my thoughts, ideas, and enjoyment of the world.

I feel a walk coming on, but I won't be competing with anyone.

Chapter 13
Exploratory Walking

"The craving for adventure can be nurtured by a hike or an exploration perhaps more than by any other activity."-- H. Dan Corbin in *Recreation Leadership*

The best scientists and explorers have the attributes of kids! They ask question and have a sense of wonder. They have curiosity. 'Who, what, where, why, when, and how!' They never stop asking questions, and I never stop asking questions, just like a five year old. –Sylvia Earle

It started with "The List." You may have a list, too. My list is of places I want to see, adventures I want to have, people I want to meet, and things I want to do before I can't anymore.

Checked off that list are two walls, the Great Wall of China and Hadrian's Wall. Hadrian's Wall was by far the greater adventure and exploration despite the fact that the Great Wall no question qualifies as more exotic and just as memorable. But we got to the Great Wall on a tour bus and I never could figure out exactly where we were except around Beijing.

Hadrian's Wall was another adventure entirely. Hadrian was Roman emperor from 117 – 138 when the Romans occupied Britain and experienced nothing but headaches. The Romans were tired of dealing with the Picts—a constant irritation, raiding the

Roman settlements in Northern England, so Hadrian ordered the troops to build a wall.

Hadrian's Wall was constructed of stone and turf across the width of Great Britain to first, prevent military raids by the Pictish tribes of Scotland to the north, and second to separate the unruly Selgovae tribe in the north from the Brigantes in the south, discouraging them from uniting. Their uniting would have meant more hair pulling and need for yet-to-be invented Advil by the occupying Romans.

Chunks of the wall still exist today. Of course, in the 2,000 years since it was built, weather, time, and farmers needing rocks have left only rubble in most places. Still there are places in the north of England where you can imagine what an impressive structure it must have been. I had to see it.

Major exploration just about always involves going somewhere beyond stepping out the front door. This was no exception. Sometimes getting to the place you want to explore is more of an adventure than the exploration itself. My "exploration" of Hadrian's Wall is a prime example. My wife and I were taking the train back to London from Edinburgh on April 20,1994. I had studied a map and saw that Hadrian's Wall, what remains of it anyway, runs across England at approximately the border between

England and Scotland. If we got off the train at Newcastle, we could probably easily get to Hadrian's Wall. Well, silly me.

I asked when we bought the train tickets at Edinburgh if we could get off the train at Newcastle and take a later one without penalty. The ticket master paused a while, scratched his head, hemmed and hawed, then replied, "I suppose so, as long as you continue the same day." Such an outlandish question may never have been asked before.

My wife, 11 years later, finally forgave me for the adventure and exploration that followed. Only a small part of this adventure involved walking, but as you will see, it was an integral part.

We got off the train with our luggage when it stopped in Newcastle. It was 11:30 am. The Information Booth lady told us the different ways to get to Hadrian's Wall. "You could rent a car (not an option in England what with their driving on the wrong side of the road), or take a cab" replied the nice lady in the booth. (How much would a cab cost?) "But if you take the train, the most direct route is through Haltwhistle. You can take a Northern Line train to Haltwhistle and then a bus to Greenhead and the Roman Army Museum."

She handed me a schedule and we went out to the train platform to wait. That train would not be along for a half hour. The schedule of the trains leaving Newcastle for London said the last train was 7:25 pm. That meant we had eight hours. Keep those eight hours in mind: they are important.

We got the train to Haltwhistle and then the bus. The bus trip from Haltwhistle to Greenhead was interesting, since we saw a part of England with the extensive farmland and hedgerows that few people except those who live there ever see.

By the time we got to Greenhead it was about 2:00 pm. Well, we got to Greenhead and then some. We had told the bus driver where we needed to get off when we got on the bus, but he had a friend of his riding with him and was engrossed in conversation. We saw Greenhead come and we expected he would stop. He didn't. His mind was in the middle of a conversation and already mentally in Carlisle, the end of the line.

After we had gone a quarter-mile down the road I asked him if that wasn't Greenhead we had just blinked and passed. He slammed on the brakes, opened the door and let us out. Now we got to walk a quarter mile back up the road. I did mention that it was chilly, didn't I? Maybe I didn't, but it was.

When we got off the bus I remembered we had not eaten lunch. Not a problem, I thought, we can stop at the pub that's right there, across the street. I walked in and was curtly informed that they were closed until 5 pm. In London and in Edinburgh, pubs stay open all the time, but in wee places such as Greenhead they follow the old dicta and close in the afternoons.

"There's a chip shop [convenience store] in Haltwhistle," he volunteered. Not an option, of course.

We started trudging up the 9 percent grade hill to the Roman Army Museum—another half hour.

Fortunately when we got to the Roman Army museum, about 2:30, the snack shop was open. Of course all they had was muffins and tea. At that point, muffins and tea sounded delicious.

Now we were there! Hadrian's Wall. The Maginot Line that mostly worked, at least better than the 20th Century version.

But Hadrian's Wall wasn't just a few steps across the street from the Roman Army Museum. It was another quarter-mile walk.

"Just walk out the door, up the road, through the gate into the sheep pasture, then climb the hill," explained the lady at the desk.

"Through the sheep pasture?" I queried incredulously.

We walked down the road, through the gate, and into the sheep pasture. It was somebody's farm. Don't they care? Can anybody just walk across their farm?

The sheep were none too pleased to see us and ran off when we came near.

We climbed the hill and there it was—a mostly well placed pile of rocks that stretches for miles and miles across the English countryside, the wall that the emperor Hadrian had built to keep the marauding Picts out of the Romans' misery.

It was fun! We climbed on the wall. We took pictures. We walked on the wall where we could. We admired the vast vistas of Northumbrian countryside. Then we toured the Roman Army Museum and watched the movie. Now it was about 4:00 pm and time to go.

Remember, the buses run only once an hour.

We started walking back down the hill with our luggage in plenty of time to catch the bus. About halfway down we saw the bus heading for Haltwhistle. It was early. About halfway down we saw the bus heading for Haltwhistle. No way would he see us if we waved our arms or hear us if we yelled, and even if he did, most likely he wouldn't stop. There was no point in running; we couldn't have even come close to catching it.

We and our luggage started walking back down the hill in plenty of time to catch the bus. About halfway down we saw the bus heading for Haltwhistle. It was early. Remember I said it was chilly? Well, it was chillier now. But we got to admire the countryside and look at some stone houses and look at the English flora in the hillside.

I was more concerned about the time, though. The bus wouldn't get there until after 5:15. That would mean we would get into Haltwhistle about 6:00. The train from Haltwhistle to Newcastle takes only 45 minutes to an hour, and the last train to London leaves at 7:25. We can make it with time to spare! I hope. If nothing out of the ordinary happens.

What if the bus breaks down? What if the train is late? What if we make the last train and the ticket master in Edinburgh scratched the wrong part of his head and told us wrong and we had to pay again? We had an hour to stand around and think about that, too.

The bus came as it was supposed to. We rode the bus to Haltwhistle—uneventfully. We found our way to the Haltwhistle train station and waited. The train would leave at about 6:10, meaning it would arrive in Newcastle about 7:10, we hoped.

Whew, we arrived in Newcastle in plenty of time and sat and waited for the last London train. While we were waiting we heard something that we will remember as long as we remember climbing Hadrian's Wall, the woman who announced the trains in Newcastle. She sang, or chanted, the train arrivals and departures.

In the mists of the quarter century since neither my wife nor I can remember exactly what she sounded like, but it was one of the most magical things we had ever heard--if only we had had a way to record her voice. But that was at least a decade before smartphones became ubiquitous.

A few years ago I called the Newcastle train station and someone there remembered the lady with the magical voice, but she has been gone from her job for some time.

Our train, the last train of the day, arrived, we got on, plopped ourselves in a seat and waited anxiously for the conductor. He spent a long time looking at our tickets, scratched his head, hemmed and hawed. After all, we had bought them early in the morning in Edinburgh and now we were sitting on a train that would arrive late in the evening in London. He punched the tickets and went on his way still scratching his head.

The train arrived at Kings Cross station at 11:33 pm along with our sigh of relief.

We still have the vivid memories of Hadrian's Wall, Northumberland, and the train announcer at Newcastle. I have been forgiven for the adventure and the subject of other walls to visit has even come up.

What walls are left to explore? I can't think of any, but they may well be waiting to enter my consciousness.

Every exploration, though, need not be so extensive or require transportation to begin it. I regularly explore on walks. It isn't some major undertaking or even planned. It's more like, "wait, I've never been over there. I wonder where it goes." Then I find out. I know of a few instances where it has provided me with a new route to follow, new things to see, and more things to pique my curiosity.

I treated myself to one particular exploration a few months ago as I wondered if the wash I was walking in went to the state park across the highway. Well, actually, it's under the highway, and because of that makes it easier to get to. That morning I didn't want to spend the extra time it would take to completely explore across the highway to the state park, but I had to see if the route I took got me there. It did. I satisfied my curiosity but I didn't finish exploring. One day soon.

But there's far more to explore.

One day I passed a man sitting on a bench in our neighborhood. It was the second day in a row I had seen him there. I remarked as I passed that I had seen him there yesterday, to which he replied, "It's my route." I have thought about that more times than I can count since then. Obviously his "route" works for him, but it would never satisfy my curiosity. I got to thinking of all the things I would have missed if I had "a route." It has to do with walking for a completely different reason than mine—exercise, head down, eyes on Fitbit, getting those steps in. Nothing wrong with that if it works, but I haven't seen that man since, so apparently having a "route" is no guarantee of sticking with walking.

The thing that came to mind immediately is "the bench." The Tucson area has what are called washes that take water safely away from structures that could wash away. In fact, neighborhoods are designed around washes. They can vary from 10-foot-wide concreted-in water tracks to quarter-mile wide wild, fully vegetated areas such as are near my house. For the most part, there are no easy ways to get to a wash with a vehicle. Sometimes there are private drives and city and county easements that enter the wash, but almost never a public roadway or dirt road that will accommodate a vehicle. That's why I thought the bench was so interesting.

This bench is heavy. It is mostly cast iron with what are left of wooden slats on the seat and the seat back completely off. The first time I saw it, the seat back was on the ground behind the bench. I laid it on the bench so it rested against the cast iron back. The bench would require a finalist in World's Strongest Man to carry it alone, what with all the iron. Two or three people could carry it, but its size and structure would make carrying it awkward. What made the abandoned bench so interesting is that it sat in a wash at least one quarter mile from any vehicle access point and that has a locked gate. Thus, when I discovered the bench, I immediately wondered how it possibly could have gotten there. Every man I mention the bench to finds it fascinating, but when I told my wife, she said something to the effect of "that's nice." How can you not find a misplaced bench, one that could have gotten where it was only with considerable difficulty, old and crusty or not, "nice"?

But it gets more interesting, yet. One day the bench had moved. It had levitated itself, or been carried, up a to a spot four feet above the level of the wash. What would prompt it to levitate or someone to move it?

Occasionally, I sit on the bench when I take that walking route or just check to see if it's still there from a route that goes close by. The spot is idyllic, surrounded by nature, and peaceful with no traffic noise and rarely people with their dogs. I can just sit there to let the world soak in. Then, sometimes I continue up a small rise to a county conservation area to continue my walk. And no, the bench cannot have arrived from there, either. It is a path that is not obvious and even less accessible by vehicle.

Of course, I never would have discovered the bench if I had not explored the wash where it sits. Getting to the wash requires walking down the hill in a neighborhood I wouldn't object to living in and past a back yard that I marvel at every time I see it. The yard is about an acre, completely enclosed by a wall, with enough trees so it is always in the shade, grass on the ground, something unusual here because most yards have rocks or paved patios, and with several fountains that contribute to the aura of a spot you would never want to leave. Had I not explored, I never would have seen this yard.

And there's more to explore. You get to one wash after walking down a dirt common area beside this idyllic yard. At that point, at least four options open up, and I have explored all of them. After all, I need to explore. One direction after a half mile or so, in the one I mentioned above that goes under the highway to the state park. Before the route to the park, a paved ramp allows access to city vehicles to do whatever they do in the wash. The top of the ramp connects with a bike and walking path, something I explored one day. Turn left and go a little farther in the wash and another part of the route goes by "the bench" eventually further around to where I can get back to my neighborhood. That's not to leave out the other direction that takes you by a shopping area at least a half mile away. These are all walks that I save for when I plan to walk farther than usual, because each route is one-and-a-half times to twice as long as my more-traveled routes.

Then there are the stairs. I had never gone down that street. After all, it dead ends (for cars anyway), so I saw no reason to walk a block down just to turn around and come back. But one day I saw someone walk out from the end of the street from a path next to the last house. I had to see what was there. That's when I discovered the path. Stairs made from four-by-six weather-resistant wood installed by the subdivision's landscapers go down to the path also maintained by the subdivision. I was so excited! I have treasured that find ever since. It has opened up endless places to explore, places I default to on my walks, places that let me enjoy the day and the entire walk always with some new place to check out.

And to think, if I restricted myself to "my route," all the things I would have missed, all the experiences I would never have had, all the things I would never have had to write about. If we had been satisfied to look out the window of the train back to London, we would never have even considered experiencing the adventure and exploring Hadrian's Wall. If I didn't have "a list" we also might not have experienced one of the best adventures in our lives.

"We do less exploring as we grow up, simply because the urge to explore wanes," wrote Nikolaas Tinbergen. Maybe for you Nikolaas. I guess I haven't grown up. I walk for the experience and to work, but I never stop asking questions "just like a five year old," as Sylvia Earle mentioned at the beginning of this chapter. Exploration is rarely the reason I head out for a walk, though it always waits patiently, eager to inspire me to see something new. Often the results of my exploratory drive are my most memorable walks. I can remember myriad walks when the occasion arises, but ones I treasure are those where I saw or experienced something new and/or unexpected. Best of all, I feel a walk coming on.

Curiosity is natural to the soul of man and interesting objects have a powerful influence on our affections.—Daniel Boone

Chapter 13.75
Hiking

When I told my son-in-law, Nate, I was writing this book, he asked, "What about hiking?" How could I have missed that? You see, he and my daughter Laurel hike, and not just walk-around-the-park hikes. They have done hikes that put our "exploration" to Hadrian's Wall to shame. For example, their six-day hike in the Spanish Pyrenees from town to town is far more impressive and enviable. Laurel describes it as a triangle-shaped route that wasn't all that hard. She wanted to keep walking. To be sure, she has nothing but admiration for people she has met who walked the trail across Spain, France, and Italy.

Nate's question deserves a little exploration of its own. After all, he and Laurel hike for many of the reasons that I go for walks.

When I was a Boy Scout oh so many years ago, we went on hikes. Maybe the rationale behind taking a bunch of 11 and 12-year-old boys on hikes is to say that you did it and to wear them out. That age boy has an excess of energy that wants channeling into something that might be considered productive or at least energy-expending.

I remember putting on "sturdy" hiking shoes and loading up my backpack with everything I would need for the day or weekend: lunch, snacks, matches, hatchet, canteen, water purification tablets, compass, change of clothes, extra socks, raingear, gloves, warm hat, first aid kit, sunscreen, insect repellent, toilet paper, binoculars, and probably more heavy stuff, and then putting the pack on, followed by taking out some "extravagances" to lighten the load. Of course it was still too heavy, but manageable. Just the empty pack was too heavy, I thought. Those memories are not of loads of fun with the lads but of grinding out miles, often in the rain, and then becoming ecstatic when I got home to dry and warm, or at least when it stopped raining and we camped for the night. It seemed as if it always rained on hikes even on the days when it started out bright and sunny. But hope of a beautiful day springs eternal, especially in the Pacific Northwest.

Using my own interpretation of hiking, and we'll get into the dictionary definition in a minute, I thought of five possible chapters where I could discuss thoughts about hiking. But in none of them does it encompass the entire idea of a hike. I thought of "See If I Can," "Social," "Exploratory," "Contemplative," and "Ruminating." But I couldn't make any of them work to encompass a hike because a hike can be all of these at the same time.

Hiking deserves a proper discussion, because it is its own special case and can differ considerably from a walk in the park, around the mall, or even in nature near home. I give it its own three-quarters chapter.

At a loss as to how to differentiate between a walk and a hike, I went to the Oxford English Dictionary (OED) hoping for a definitive answer. A hike, it says is, "A vigorous or laborious walk; a tramp or march; a walking tour or expedition undertaken for exercise or pleasure." So that could include a walk with lots of hills. Certainly not definitive.

Under the verb definition, the OED adds "to go for a long walk." So define "long."

Look under the verb "to walk" and we find "The action or an act of travelling or moving, esp. on foot."

But think about this. Remember Foster Powell and Captain Barclay from the "Competitive Walking" chapter? When Powell and Barclay walked, they called them walks, not hikes, and we also might call them treks. We know that people went for actual hikes in the early 1800s, but those were sometimes treks through the wilderness all geared up with a supply of food and adequate clothing for any eventuality such as those John Muir took to explore Yosemite, the Grand Canyon, and the Sequoia Regions with the idea of making them national parks, and those John James Audubon took to draw the birds of America.

Those differing ideas about hikes and walks leave it up to our own definitions, all subjective. Going on a hike sounds more strenuous, but I have been on some walks that might be every bit a strenuous as some hikes, just maybe not as long. Maybe long is the key. Certainly if I were to pack up everything I would need and head out for the day, I could call that a hike. But how about half a day, or two hours? It brings to mind the passage from Alice in Wonderland that I cited in Chapter 4 on Contemplative Walking, a word "means just what I choose it to mean — neither more nor less."

My neighbor, I found out, has a looser definition of hike. We were talking one day about a particular route in the desert that I used to take before developers bulldozed 50 acres or so. He called that a hike. Calling it that never entered my mind. To him it's a hike, but to me just a walk in the desert and not a very long one at that.

We can do the same things on a hike as we can on a walk. To my way of thinking, we just have longer to do it. We can contemplate the world, ruminate ideas, see if we can, hike with another person, and certainly explore.

To get a better picture of the differences between hiking and walking, I went to Summit Hut, a store in Tucson that stocks all manner of equipment to take yourself out into the wild, enough to keep you stocked up and out of money. When we step out the door for a walk, our only requirement is a decent pair of shoes, and maybe not even that. I spoke with two avid hikers, Ray Kuhn and Taylor Brandlen at Summit Hut wanting to find out their thoughts on hiking. Just how should someone prepare for a hike?

Ray was an engineer in a previous life, and came to work at Summit Hut after he ended his 35-year career. He told me his most memorable hike was the one he took with Taylor Brandlen to the summit of Mt. Whitney, the tallest mountain in the contiguous United States at 14,505 feet, 14,508 feet, 14,491 feet or 14,497 feet depending on who's measuring. Regardless, it's tall and the 14-foot possible difference in measurement doesn't affect the exertion required to climb it. It took two days plus a day or two to get acclimated to the altitude.

Taylor has hiked the Grand Canyon rim-to-rim 24 times. I made him confirm that number. That's rim to rim, 21.4 miles, down then up, one way. He's also hiked the 800-mile long Arizona Trail, Mexico border to Utah border, which includes a rim-to-rim Grand Canyon trek on the way from the south.

The Arizona Trail was his first major hike. He hesitated to admit his inexperience to hikers he met along the way, fearful that they would think he had picked the easiest of the long-distance US trails and could be considered not to be a "real" hiker for choosing it. To me walking 800 miles is nothing to be hesitant to admit to. Many of the folks he met along the way were experienced long-distance hikers who had done other of the long trails. They told him that the Arizona Trail was every bit as hard or harder than the Appalachian or Pacific Crest Trails.

What I particularly wanted to know from the hiking experts at Summit Hut was about special equipment requirements and considerations for a hike. After all, a wilderness hike involves going lots farther than a walk around the neighborhood so incurs the possibility of creating untold misery with improper preparation.

Curious about hiking poles, I wanted to know if they actually helped on a hike. I have seen people using them and wondered if they were simply an affectation designed to make someone look like a "real" hiker. Ray told me that they were particularly helpful going downhill because they took stress off knees. You put part of your weight on the poles and that eases the knee strain. I also wondered about carrying them because I certainly would want to have to deal with a long pole when I didn't need one. They telescope, like the legs on a camera tripod, so fit tidily into a pack. He added that the store rents them out.

Not surprisingly, both Ray and Taylor said the most important piece of equipment is shoes. They say shoes can help make a hike a glorious experience or doom it to utter misery depending on the shoes and their fit. Fitting hiking shoes is a unique system because it accounts for how well the shoes will work on a hike, something considerably different than buying running shoes or shoes to wear to work.

For example, Taylor told me that he wears a size 10 ½ shoe in daily life but a size 13 shoe for a hike. Why in a minute. How they measure shoes is an essential consideration. They measure not just heel to toe, but also heel to ball, then find the shoe that fits best for both those measurements. Where someone's arch meets up with the arch in the shoe is just as important as making sure the shoe is long enough. And that might require trying on several different pairs, and not just for toe and arch placement.

Taylor's size-13 hiking shoe is a case in point. A shoe where toes jam up against the toe of the shoe can ruin a perfect, or even a just enjoyable, hike. That's a vital consideration especially going downhill where a foot sliding forward in shoes can result in a bruised toe nail even to the point of losing a nail. That means walking with difficulty, and naturally no hiking for the months it takes for the nail to regrow. Taylor's size 13 shoe avoids that problem because his toes never hit the toe of the shoes. A determining factor, of course, is the heel to ball measurement.

In other chapters I wrote about how a walk can restore inner peace, refresh our brains, and correct Directed Attention Fatigue.

A hike provides a huge opportunity for all that because we are out of the clatter, hustle and bustle of the world. Successconsciousness.com provides what I think is an excellent description, "Inner peace means among other things that there is no overthinking and too much analyzing of every situation. It means no running from one thought to another, constantly ruminating about some past incident, no constant dwelling on hurts and what people said or did. It means no waste of time, energy and attention on unimportant and meaningless thoughts." Turning off thinking, especially thinking that goes in directions we don't want it to go, creates an experience that for me, at least, doesn't come along that often. Taylor describes his mind as going in a similar direction.

He reported a calming of his mind on his four-week hike of the Arizona Trail. The first two weeks it raced with the usual memories, obsessions, and concerns that many of us face when left alone to our own thoughts. But something interesting happened after those two weeks, his brain just turned off "unimportant and meaningless thoughts," much like we do during meditation.

And that's one of the main reasons Taylor hikes, for the opportunity to get meditative introspection. What works for him is going out on a hike alone and ending up at a secluded spot to sit and think, to get his head together.

Taylor has two pieces of what I thought was great advice: "hike your own hike" and "stay alive, have fun, and keep walking." Don't let anyone else push you into hiking somewhere you won't or can't enjoy, or doesn't accomplish for you what you want from a hike, or somehow entice you into doing something that makes you feel unsafe or uncomfortable. Just as important for me is "walk your own walk." How far and how fast I walk is entirely my decision and the goal of the walk should be my own, not anyone else's such as the guilt because the walk was too short or too slow. We'll look at guilt walking in the next chapter.

We can call a walk a hike if we want and call a hike a walk if we want. So go for a walk or a hike and contemplate, ruminate, see if you can, take someone with you if you want, and by all means explore.

I feel a walk, or hike, coming on.

Chapter 14
Guilt Walking

Mark Twain is supposed to have said that golf was "a good walk spoiled." He didn't, as it happens; the first mention of the quote was in a 1948 *Saturday Evening Post* article. It has been attributed to Leon Wilson, a couple named the Allens, and William Gladstone more credibly than to Mark Twain. Regardless, the statement is celebrated and oft-repeated. The same judgment could be decreed for the step counter, or pedometer, something Mark Twain, or another person of his time could not have even imagined. I believe a walk should be an adventure, an event where I enjoy the world around me, a time when I get new ideas and flesh out old ones. A step counter can be, and sometimes ends up as, "a good walk spoiled."

Yes, I walk about 25 miles a week, and the only reason I know is that I have a step counter. My step counter only counts steps and figures how far and how long I've walked. Other step counters go all the way and almost keep track of your entire life. A Fitbit, for example, can, among other things, log food, share your stats, monitor heart rate, track GPS, track sleep, notify of calls and texts, track how long it takes to do something, pair with apps, remind you to charge it, in addition to its primary purpose of counting steps, calories burned, and calculating distance walked and time exercised. A step counter is a purveyor of guilt, and guilt can spoil many a good walk.

Data, such as daily averages, I can figure out myself and do my own calculations if I want, but I don't want. "Coming up short" could spoil an entire week of walks.

Then there's the smart phone. Pair that with a Fitbit, and you get the full disaster. Here's the opportunity to pitch yourself untold guilt, keeping track of everything and telling the world about your successes or (gasp) failures. Trouble is, the Health App on the iphone doesn't even calculate correctly. With my step counter, I set the length of my step, 32 inches, and it calculates the distance I walked from that. But there's no way to set the step length with the Health App. Just curious, I figured out what it was once, but now can't remember exactly except it was in the mid-20 inches. Yes, I could figure out the real distance from that, but why should I have to? Then there's "Map My Walk," the complete disaster that stops mid walk because apparently it loses the GPS. More about that in Chapter 15 on Exercise.

I got my simple step counter for information, but then it gradually and seductively took control. Guilt rears its head if I don't walk "enough," if I don't get my 25 miles in during a week. Then because I need to walk to "catch up," I may overdo. The information I bought it for ended up creating guilt and ruling my walks, sometimes ruining my enjoyment of them.

Forget to put it on and you beat yourself up because you didn't "get credit" for the walk, as if a machine can give you credit. But worse, a Fitbit can give credit and report you to a website where you share your exercise and so have guilt pitched twice because you forgot to put it on.

Fitbit's official website promises, "Use the Fitbit app to share a view or a selfie once you've reached the peak of your workout. Your pic and stats can be sent to friends and followers on any social channel, or through email and text." How special, post it to Facebook for everyone to see. Even more, you can "Challenge Friends & Family. Stay encouraged to move more by using your steps to climb the leaderboard, or compete with friends and family in Fitbit Challenges." Wow, the guilt that can pitch. Beat yourself up because you didn't out-exercise your cousin Ruth or 80-year-old Uncle Carl.

Just wait until it gets connected to your insurance company. Oh, wait! It has, and one, as of this writing, is requiring it from new policy holders. One life insurance company only sells insurance policies that include their insureds wearing fitness trackers such as Fitbits and Apple Watches that, coupled with smartphones, can report physical activity back to the company. In addition, those people who meet "exercise targets" get gift cards and other tasty things. The insurance company figures that since people will live longer, they will pay more premiums and require fewer payouts, so it comes out ahead. Older policies are scheduled to convert.

The insurance company says that since it is so highly regulated, it won't be able to raise rates for those who don't meet goals because it has to justify "in actuarial terms" increases in policy charges. Well, duh. They already collect data from their insureds that will show that the people who exercise enough live longer and are better risks and thus those who don't exercise ought to pay higher premiums. Worldwide data on fitness tracking show that those who are tracked live 13 to 21 years longer than their more sedentary, or maybe tracking-averse insureds. Watch those premiums go up.

Look at the Apple Watch. Apple's website extols its virtues, "All kinds of health records. All in one place. View a consolidated timeline of your health history — such as lab results, immunizations, and medications. Even if the data is from different health institutions. You'll also be notified when new records are available."

But taking into consideration its awareness of privacy issues, Apple says, "The Health app lets you keep all your health and fitness information under your control and in one place on your device. You decide which information is placed in Health and which apps can access your data through the Health app. [Sure you do. Look at Google's promises of privacy.] . . . Your health data stays up to date across all your devices automatically using iCloud, where it is encrypted while in transit and at rest." But what if your health insurance company offers discounts for keeping them up to date, just as they do for people who put a device in their cars to monitor their driving as the insurance companies have begun doing?

Its gets even worse. My personal trainer's wife works for a company that provides Fitbits to employees so they can keep track of how much exercise their employees get. If the employee meets specific goals, he or she receives an extra $400 a month. Sounds good, and who wouldn't want an extra $400 a month? But wait. It's voluntary now, but employers want to ensure that their employees are able not only to get to work but to be effective at work, so look for the "voluntary" part to go ever so stealthily by the wayside. Johanna Mischke, Editor-in-Chief at Wearable Technologies wrote, that "The healthcare space is going through a digital revolution with the invasion of technology. Medical wearables with artificial intelligence and big data are providing an added value to healthcare with a focus on diagnosis, treatment, patient monitoring and prevention." Oh, the Pollyanna outlook.

Wearable devices can track worker productivity along with monitoring their "wellbeing." Old hat are the devices that count computer keystrokes of employees. Now added are monitoring if their employees are not getting enough exercise, feeling a little poorly, suffering a hangover, or otherwise not up to snuff. And the employer will do the deciding what needs to be addressed.

The market for wearables is huge. GlobalData suggests in a report that by 2023, the wearables market will double to some $54 billion annually.

Guilt, guilt, guilt. What better way to motivate is there to "get that walk in"? Lots of better ways. Trouble is, in the case of letting a pedometer dictate my walk, I'm not walking for the enjoyment but to assuage the guilt. Then there's the dread: Insurance rates go up because I don't exercise enough; I won't get the bonus every month; my boss will know if I drank too much last night; or, the company might see an "irregularity" and decide I'm too big a risk.

This isn't the guilt that haunts for doing something such as robbing a bank, cheating on a spouse, keeping the money in a found wallet while putting the cleaned-out wallet in the mailbox. Rather it is disappointment with self for not doing enough. That can be a powerful motivator, but that guilt can also have the effect of throwing a damper on success and conditioning.

Maud Purcell, LCSW, CEAP wrote in an article on psychcentral.com "The truth, however, is that guilt is the greatest destroyer of emotional energy. It leaves you feeling immobilized in the present by something that has already occurred." After a while, we can get the feeling that since we aren't meeting our fitness "goals," we are failing. What's the point in keeping on beating ourselves up. Just quit that walking stuff.

And it gets even worse, yet. Guilt saps strength. Here's a demonstration you can do yourself that shows the physical effect of negative emotions. Unless you've seen it done or experienced it yourself, you won't believe it. I used to do this demonstration for my college classes. It is not original with me; I read about it or heard about it on motivational tapes many years ago, though I can't remember the source or sources. No doubt there are several. Two students came to the front of the room. One was the pushee, the other one, the pusher. I had the pushee hold out his or her arm and say something like "I can play the piano well." It doesn't matter if he or she could; just saying it is enough. Then I had the other student, the pusher, try to push down the arm of the test student. Often the pusher couldn't or had a great deal of difficulty pushing the arm down.

Next I had the pushee say something like "I can't play the piano" while holding out his or her arm. The pusher was able to easily push down the arm of the test student. No one in the class could believe what they had just seen. The two students switched sides—same result. Because the class would figure that I wasn't entirely honest and just wanted to prove a point, I never acted as the pusher or pushee myself.

Guilt has an even more negative effect on strength than just thinking we can't do something. Giving control of walking to a machine can result in guilt. Even not walking for a day or so can result in guilt. The more guilt, the more it saps strength. A negative emotion is far more debilitating than one negative thought.

The reasons for a walk that keep me looking forward to it rather than thinking of it as duty enfold the pleasures it will give me or the things I will accomplish, the pleasure of seeing the world, exploring, getting ideas, working out how to approach a piece of writing, or just enjoying the day. But, the step counter is patient. It religiously keeps track (as long as I have it on), so it can make sure I have walked "enough." And it sends out invisible waves making me check to see how I did. And if I haven't walked enough? That's when it tries to wheedle itself into my psyche. I find myself making up 100 or 200 steps before bed so I have "enough" or bump over to the next thousand.

Still, there are ways that people lessen the chance of their step counters and Fitbits pitching guilt. I'll look at some of those in the next chapter, "Exercise Walking." If those work, great, they provide a reason for walking that isn't exclusively exercise. The truth is, if someone does anything only for the exercise, chances are, he or she won't continue.

As I wrote in Chapter 1, a walk "can be the highlight of the day, the activity you wake up in the morning thinking about, the plan you make for your daily adventure." "Getting those steps in" works for a while, but just as with an exercise program, its motivation wears out and guilt can set in. I want a walk to make me feel joy and to get my ideas and thoughts in order if it is to be a proper walk.

As I wrote in Chapter 8, "The Productivity Trap," "The problem is that I get so caught up in the numbers, the 'progress,' that those numbers, that progress becomes more important and the reason I have for walking gets overshadowed by averages and standard deviations and deciding if I have walked 'enough.' Then, when I do better than average, I can pat myself on the back and tell myself, 'good work.' Yes, it is 'good work,' but the real question is am I gaining on accomplishing what it will take to get my brain where I want it to go?" As I quoted Taylor Brandlen saying in the Hiking Chapter, "Hike your own hike," or in this case, "walk your own walk."

I feel a completely guilt-free walk coming on.

Chapter 15
Exercise Walking, the one-half reason

Credit (or blame) goes to the ancient Babylonians for New Year's resolutions. Every year at their 12-day New Year celebration in mid-March they called Akitu, they made resolutions. Though we can't know for sure what they resolved, the cuneiform records say they made their resolutions in the form of promises to the gods that they would give back those things they borrowed and pay their debts. Possibly they made other resolutions that they never recorded. It almost certainly wasn't to walk more since that was just about the only way people got around, and more exercise was not an issue with farmers, the vast majority. Maybe the tradesmen thought about getting more exercise, but even they usually carried goods on their backs, if they didn't use a donkey, and walked to wherever they were going. No matter what the resolutions, though, scary consequences ensued if they didn't keep them such as failed crops and even the snuffing out of their existence.

The New Year's Resolution tradition has stuck these thousands of years. In fact, one study, "Auld Lang Syne" by J.C. Norcross et al reported that 40 to 45 percent of Americans make one or more resolutions every year and intend to accomplish them, at least when they make the resolutions. But our failing to keep the resolutions results in nowhere near the dire consequences the Babylonians imagined. People sometimes make resolutions because of guilt. They feel guilty about their misbehaviors of the previous 12 months, or 12 years, and resolve to correct them and their results. One of the top two resolutions is to "get more exercise." The other one to "eat better." The way they are worded destines these resolutions to failure, though. We'll look at why that is in a little while. In the meantime, we'll look at two dirty little secrets.

One of the ways people resolve to "get more exercise" is by walking. Dirty little secret one is even though walking is good exercise, if people do it for exercise, before long they won't. It has to do with intentions. We intend to do something. Intention always precedes exercise even if it's by five minutes. Intentions drive walking and exercise. If we don't intend, we don't exercise. Walking, what this book is about, is good exercise, but as we will see, if exercise is the only reason for a walk, chances are after a while, you won't walk.

Here's why. Intentions change, and what we intended to do changes to something else. As it happens, that's dirty little secret two. For example, Gold's Gym says its traffic jumps 40 percent in December and January every year. But since those good intentions change, their dirty little secret is that the gym industry depends on intentions changing. Planet Fitness, for example, reports that half of its members never do more than drive by their gyms, possibly feeling guilty and thinking "when I have time. . .," but never stopping in. It's a good thing, too, because their average gym holds about 300 people but they may sign up 6,000 on year-long contracts.

It's possible that the very situation of gyms is what keeps people away. I know it does me. I don't like them. Going is too much trouble. I have to get ready to go by changing clothes then driving there. When I get there, the gym can be crowded or empty; it doesn't matter. I am not particularly sociable and I don't want to wait to use equipment. I can do just about all the exercises the gym equipment uses at home with free weights, stretch band, or body weight training, no changing clothes, no driving, no being sociable. I can't say for sure, but I suppose other people might have the same or similar aversions I do.

Those gym figures are easy to come by, but figures of how many people walk are all but impossible without a credible study, one that I haven't found yet. Just like the Babylonians, we intend to achieve our resolution, but unlike the Babylonians, crops won't fail and the world won't end if we don't follow through. That's most likely the reason people start with those good intentions in January to get more exercise, lose weight, and get fit, but get new intentions and abandon their resolutions before Super Bowl Sunday.

"Motivation is what gets you started. Habit is what keeps you going." Brian Tracy

Habits die hard. That's why they're called habits: they're habitual. For example, my habit in the summer, I go for a walk early, often before seven because after that, it's too hot to walk. That's my habit, but one I prefer to break because I like going for a walk later in the morning after I've settled into the day. I started the walking habit a few years ago. As I've described in other parts of this book, I've enjoyed walking my whole life, and a few years ago, I made it a habit.

I religiously kept track of every day's walk, writing it down on the form I created. But recently, I decided to give it a break. I don't walk for exercise but for other reasons, so why keep careful track of how many steps I take every day? Things got so bad that I was competing with myself, thinking I needed to walk more and more every week or I would somehow fall off the wagon and have slugdom overcome me. It's always lurking, you know. It became a contest with myself and created a guilt trip. (See chapter 14)

How Many Steps?

Looking back at the sheets where I kept track (yes, I used paper rather than Excel), I see that many weeks I walked more than 30 miles. (If I had used Excel, I would have been tempted to use all the nifty Excel tools to calculate "how I did" on my walks with medians, means, standard deviations, p-values and anything else that might enable me to waste time looking at data that means nothing. Think of the guilt I could have pitched myself then.) But I got to wondering why that far. Coming up with no good answer, a few months ago I decided to just walk 25 miles a week, 49,500 of my steps. But why 25 miles? Why not 20 miles, 22 ½ miles, or 30 miles? No good reason. The step counter insidiously took over my walking and the reasons I walked. I forgot to ask if walking was doing what I wanted it to do, getting ideas and enjoying the world. So I took a break, for a while, at least, not from walking but from religiously keeping track of steps. That brings up the question of how many steps is enough, and am I walking "enough"?

The mantra, ever since 1964 when that Japanese company invented a step counter and called it 10,000 Step Meter (in Japanese), the more ingenuous and intellectually lazy of the news media have sucked into that number.

Catrine Tudor-Locke and David R. Bassett Jr. have come up with an answer, saying it is based on "currently available evidence," evidence they don't cite. They classify daily walking steps for adults into categories of sedentary (fewer than 5,000), low active (5,000-7499), somewhat active (7500-9999), and active (more than 10,000). Then they leave a super-person category of highly active for people who walk more than 12,500 steps a day.

In spite of their classifications, though they later admit that they have no direct evidence that any number of steps results in any reduction in mortality. They even go so far as to cite what Dr. Yoshiro Hatano said to the American College of Sports Medicine in 2001 that the 10,000 steps mantra arose from a marketing gimmick of Yamasa Corporation that made pedometers and encouraged Japanese walking clubs to follow that lead. The reason for the 10,000 steps mantra, though, they admit is that "it is simple, easy to remember, and provides people with a concrete goal."

Of course, walking 10,000 steps may have a number of health benefits such as less body fat and lower blood pressure, but that is an arbitrary goal. Why not 11,000 steps or 9,000? In fact, what exactly is the difference between 9650 steps and 10,000 other than 350? If someone walks those 350 extra steps will he or she suddenly transform into an "active" person as opposed to "somewhat active"? Does an early death await that 9650-step person that the 10,000-step person won't have? Many people simply can't walk 10,000 steps—five miles—a day for a couple of reasons. One, it can take the better part of two hours to walk that far, and if someone works eight hours a day, an hour for lunch, has a commute of even one hour total, and there's still time that needs to be set aside for such mundane activities as eating, family time, and personal errands. Two, some people simply are not in good enough condition to walk five miles in a day, though they may be able to build up to it. I know I don't have either the time or inclination to walk five miles every day, even though I am physically able to do it.

There are some people whose situation does allow them to get 10,000 steps in. They can walk at lunch, walk between offices at their work, walk across parking lots by parking farther away from the door to the store, and generally make a point of walking as much as possible. It does require thinking about it and planning. But they are in an enviable position compared to lots of working people whose entire work day is behind a desk in a cubicle.

I can't help it, though. I have a lingering guilt, doubt, or curiosity as I wrote about in the "Guilt Walking" Chapter (14). Did I walk enough? So I came up with a new way to measure: walk just as far as the new ideas continue. I have noticed that ideas do stop at a some point in a walk with my mind going into less productive and often unpleasant places. I don't want to stop before the ideas run out, and I don't see any real reason to walk more than that except for the nagging problem that I'm usually nowhere near home when the ideas give up on me, but it's not the same distance every time. I can't break the habit of the step counter, though. Maybe later.

This chapter is about exercise, though. I can't say with any certainty why most people walk, but an article in *WalkingInfo*, "General Pedestrian Statistics" said that 27 percent of people walk for exercise. A distant second was personal errands at 17.3 percent and a third of recreation at 15.3 percent. Of course, that's how all the articles in the newspapers and magazine approach walking, exercise. And yes, walking is good for you, no question. It will make you feel better. It can help you lose weight, though that's mostly wishful thinking, and something we'll look at next. It strengthens the heart. It helps you think better. It strengthens bones. It alleviates depression. It reduces the risks of breast and colon cancer. It improves fitness. It improves physical functions. All those benefits are more or less common knowledge.

That second dirty little secret: if exercise is the only reason to walk, chances are people won't keep it up because, as mentioned earlier, intentions and resolutions change and old habits skulk back. And many of those who encourage walking do so disingenuously. They suggest that walking will make us lose weight. In almost every situation, that's simply not true. My wife even picked up a *Prevention* book at the checkout stand of the grocery store entitled "Walk Off Weight." She saw it and immediately thought of my book and me. The book goes into some detail about what to do to "Transform Your Body" by walking.

The book's not just about walking but some ancillary things that can affect or improve walking, so the title was simply a marketing gimmick. It talks about "sidestepping roadblocks" that gobble up time and motivation for exercise. It describes how to drop "Two Sizes in 6 Weeks." It adds tummy tightening exercises. Not nearly done, it provides a solution for stress and suggests walking stretches and "power foods." Finally, it talks about better posture. One chapter busts some walking myths, which we'll get into in a minute.

Weight Loss

Shedding pounds requires more than going for a walk around the neighborhood. In fact one study "Increasing daily walking lowers blood pressure in postmenopausal women" by Kerrie Moreau and others found that after a 24-week program of walking the women's blood pressure dropped slightly but neither their weight nor body mass index (BMI) did. Here's why.

In order to lose one pound, we have to burn a net 3500 calories. A 140-pound person, for example, burns 223 calories an hour walking three miles per hour, about a mile every 20 minutes. A 200-pound person burns 319 calories. Put more memorably, eat a 540-calorie Big Mac and you would need to walk an hour and 43 minutes to burn it off. Add a Super-Sized Coke and fries to that and it would take seven hours to burn it off. That is in addition to the 15 hours it would take a 140-pound person and the 11 hours it would take a 200-pound person to burn off one pound without the Big Mac and Coke. Even a week of a 200-pound person walking, assuming walking the two-and-a-half hours (30 minutes a day, five days a week that the medical profession mantra encourages) would burn not even 800 calories. Even walking seven hours a week, an hour a day, every day, would only burn 2233 calories. That's still a far cry from the 3500 calories required to lose a pound.

The intensity of exercise determines how many calories someone burns off. Heart rate is the most accurate measure of intensity. For example, a 50-year-old 180-pound man walking with a heart rate of 90 beats per minute, burns 401calories an hour. Bump that heart rate up to 120 beats per minute and the same person burns 673 calories an hour. Older people burn proportionately more calories at the same heart rate than do their younger peers. In a week, the 673 calories add up to over 4700 calories, enough to burn a pound of fat, but remember, that has to be net calories to lose a pound. And 120 beats per minute is hard work for some people, maybe even impossible, not just an easy stroll.

One reason for age being a factor is that the maximum recommended heart rate decreases by age. We are supposed to subtract our age from 220 and multiply by 90 percent to get our maximum heart rate. Thus, a 25-year-old would have a maximum heart rate of 175 while a 70-year-old a maximum heart rate of 135. That of course, manufactured the need for heart rate monitors, often included with step counters such as FitBit, to calculate exercise intensity of calories burned. But heart rate monitors are notoriously inaccurate. Several consumer studies such as one by Kaiser Permanente have found that the chest monitors outperform the wrist monitors for accuracy, and my own experience confirms that. Even those can be off by considerable numbers. I have had issues with the chest monitor where I have had it read 170-plus beats per minute (someone would have needed to call the paramedics), but when I felt my pulse, my heart is obviously beating at under 100 beats per minute. I have learned to say, "yeah right" to an obviously inaccurate reading or not bother with the monitor at all, the case now.

The Borg Scale

I don't know where and could not find where these calculations for recommended heart rate originated, and their accuracy depends not only the age of the individual but on the physical condition. Heart rate is important, though. Which brings up the Borg Scale, an easier way to measure and understand heart rate and without any devices. Gunnar Borg, of Stockholm University in Sweden, in January 1962 came up with a way to subjectively measure exercise intensity. His scale, now widely used by physical training folks, rates intensity of exercise by perceived intensity, the Rate of Perceived Exertion (RPE). His original scale went from 6, essentially not moving, to 20 "maximal exertion," why in a moment. Later he revised it to go from 0 to 10. Explaining his original scale, he reported in his 1982 paper "Psychophysical bases of perceived exertion" that the perceived intensity as reported by the person exercising corresponded relatively accurate that person's heart rate multiplied by 10. Thus, if someone had a perceived intensity of 12, his or her heart rate would be somewhere around 120. Calculating it this way makes the measurement more applicable to the individual for measuring every aspect of his or her physical activity, than, say, general mantra to walk 30 minutes a day, five days a week or calculate calories burned by amount of time exercised. Here's the original scale.

#	Level of Exertion
6	No exertion at all
7	
7.5	Extremely light (7.5)
8	
9	Very light
10	
11	Light
12	
13	Somewhat hard
14	
15	Hard (heavy)
16	
17	Very hard
18	
19	Extremely hard
20	Maximal exertion

Borg Scale of Rating of Perceived Exertion

One thing that the exercise-for-weight-loss people commonly leave out, though, is the residual increased metabolism after we end a workout, "afterburn." And this part is important. Depending on the intensity of a workout, "afterburn" can last 24 hours. Of course, in order to get the most burn, you have to have worked out with a degree of intensity that goes beyond a recreational stroll. One website suggests that eating protein immediately after a workout cranks up the afterburn. But you still have to do more than mosey for a few minutes to crank it up.

The key to the amount of afterburn we can expect is the intensity of the exercise it follows. Running and jogging results in more afterburn than fast walking and far more than just the casual stroll observing the world and enjoying the outdoors that I is my wont. But then, I don't walk for exercise, either. I'm one of the 12.3 percent of people in the walking survey who walk for "other" reasons.

The Myths

The myths in the Prevention book *Walk Off Weight* I mentioned mostly repeat what I have observed already, but they bear repeating and commenting on, as if I could resist.

Myth: Walking has to be a workout. Not a chance, they point out. They quote Sarah Kusch, a Los Angeles fitness coach, who says "the trap many people fall into is always think you have to go big or go home. And if they don't have time to go for 30 or 60 minutes, then they don't go at all." That, of course, implies that people are walking solely for exercise, not for the enjoyment of the walk.

Myth: You have to hit 10,000 steps per day. Kusch points out that focusing on the number of steps can be "a big blow to motivation." As I mentioned in Chapter 14, it's letting a machine run your life.

Myth: As long as you're walking and counting calories, you can eat whatever you want to still lose weight. Well, duh. The book points out that we need a balance of nutrients including fats from avocados and olive oil, protein and carbohydrates early in the day, but not carbs from cakes, cookies, pasta and white bread. But you know the drill.

Myth: You burn a lot of calories walking, so you can eat more. We just talked about that.

Motivation, and How to Get It and Stay Motivated

I have taught goal-setting for many years in seminars and as a college instructor. I use the SMART goal system, probably the most common one. In the event you don't know, SMART is an acronym for Specific, Measurable, Achievable, Realistic, and Time Sensitive. Peter Gollwitzer added a new wrinkle he calls "Implementation Intentions." He reports that "better performances are observed when people set themselves challenging, specific goals as compared with challenging but vague goals (so-called 'do your best' goals)." Specific is more than just "walk more," "exercise more," or "eat better," because with a goal like that, just walking around the block, going to the gym twice, and forgoing a Big Mac qualify as "more" and "better."

He reports accurately and in line with the "specific" part of the SMART system that it works better because of "feedback and self-monitoring advantages." But Gollwitzer adds one handy thing to specificity, if-then. That involves adding when, where, and how to the goal. For example, "If it's Saturday at 9 AM, then I will walk one mile in the park on Main St. and if it's 9 AM every other day, then I will walk one mile in my neighborhood." A typical SMART goal would simply state something like, "I walk at least one mile every day."

That seems to make implementation of the goal a tad rigid, but Gollwitzer explains that "people can always stop the effect of implementation intentions by deliberately giving up their commitment to the respective goal intention or the implementation intention itself." That's a convoluted way of saying they made the choice of that method, so they can change it if they want. (why didn't he just say that?) Makes sense to me, but that's also why people give up on exercise. The real issue is how to keep the intentions for going for a walk working. And that's where the tactic of the gyms come in regarding people's changing intentions. Remember, much of this book is about how to enjoy the world more with a walk and free your mind to accomplish more things.

Continuing with SMART goals, the M stands for measurable. That's what step counters, Fit Bits, and Apple Watches do, among other things. Thus part of an intention to walk a specific distance, number of steps, or average heart rate comes under the category of measuring. Part of the intention could be to keep an average heart rate of 90 beats per minute or 2500, 5000, or 9650 steps a day.

Achievable can fly in the face of measurable, though. If an intention is to walk 10,000 steps a day, the achievability factor may come into question. As I mentioned earlier, it takes most of two hours to walk 10,000 steps a day, something beyond the possibility of achievement for many people. What is achievable? That's certainly up to the individual. For me, just about any number of steps could be achievable since my time is my own. Which brings us to Realistic.

Realistically, I could walk two hours every day and get 10,000 or 12,000 steps in. But it is not realistic. I have other things to do. For some people, walking even 5,000 steps a day isn't realistic since their physical condition won't allow it. As a result, setting up a specific, measurable, achievable goal of even 5,000 steps is not realistic. They might accomplish it one day or even two, but their bodies would know it's ridiculous and rebel, making any walking at all impossible or torture until the tortured body recovers, several days or even weeks depending on the overuse. They give up that "walking stuff" as a bad idea because they are "always" injured.

My own experience reinforces that idea. For several years decades ago, I was a runner. Most weeks I ran 60 miles. But I gave it up. I was always hurt. Overuse caused my Iliotibial band to become so inflamed that I could barely walk and certainly not run. The Iliotibial band is a long fascia running down the outside of the thigh that connects to the outside of the knee. Overuse or structural predisposition to the injury (my son has the same problem) can result in its becoming inflamed. In my stubbornness, I was not about to give up on running, which I believed at the time was such a benefit to me, I went to doctors, chiropractors, and physical therapists to find out how to fix myself. They were little or no help. A physical therapist told me to ice my knee after running, and that helped make it feel better, which it did, but never kept the injury at bay. Eventually, I just said "forget it." The constant injury and pain wasn't worth it. I went to riding a bicycle instead and that took care of the Iliotibial band problem. Running wasn't realistic.

Time sensitive rounds out the SMART goals. Usually that involves accomplishing something in a specific length of time. It could mean walking five miles a day or 10 miles a week, or anything else that has a time measurement. The idea is that it motivates to accomplish something within a measured time period. It can take the form of preparing for an organized walk, for example. So, if there's a five mile community walk coming up and someone wants to participate in it, the time sensitive part would be to walk enough to be able to accomplish that five-mile walk. But then what? The problem is that once a goal is achieved, there needs to be another goal to take its place or the motivation for walking disappears.

Motivation

So, in that vein, intentions change, and that change may not help exercise at all. People can stay motivated by making a game of exercise, or in this case, walking. One way is by using smart phone apps such as Map My Walk. When I went to the Walk With a Doc event, several people said they used such apps on their phones. I had to try it out. If my experience is representative, it was a waste of time. The first time I used it, Map My Walk worked and drew a nifty map of where I had walked. I believe it worked right only once. The next time, it stopped mid-walk. I got home and discovered that it had quit halfway through. I began checking on it after that and would find out that it had lost contact with the GPS or just had a spasm at various, random spots. I would restart it, but eventually I gave up on it. Using it was fun when it worked, but I have little patience with machines and software that don't work. I have mentioned it to other people, such as Taylor Brandlen and Ray Kuhn at Summit Hut, both of whom thought that Map My Walk and the other similar apps were pretty much garbage.

A way to make a game of walking, though, involves the thermometer. You know what those are. Draw a thermometer and mark how much you do, how many steps, how far, how much time, or whatever you want to measure whenever you walk. Then seeing the progress motivates continued walking. I could do that, but I see no point in it because I walk for reasons that have little or nothing to do with steps, distance or time and are thus immeasurable, unspecific, and not time sensitive. They are, however, both achievable and reasonable if I were inclined to factor those in. But without the rest of the SMART goals, they are pointless. But once again, when you reach the top of the thermometer, what then? Only another goal keeps the motivation going. And if exercise is the reason for walking, continued specific motivation is essential to keep it up.

I got to thinking about how I could word my own implementation intentions about walking, because, after all, I walk for work for mental fitness and to avoid the possible guilt of not walking "enough," at least until I can divest myself of that guilt. I have tried a couple of different things. One is to deliberately walk at a slower pace than I might normally. It's much easier to enjoy the world if I am passing it by a little slower. I can stop and look at things I hadn't seen before, such as the cholla I mentioned in Chapter 3. Then there were the red acacia seed pods I saw the other day. If I had been dutifully staring ahead to "get those steps in," I most likely would not have stopped to enjoy them. I would hurriedly have passed them by intent on the exercise, missing out on a memorable walk and experience.

Exercise is only the half reason for walking, for me, anyway. I can soak in the day, listen to nature, watch nature, get terrific ideas and analyze maybe even more things than I need to, but benefit nonetheless. I can take walks that I will remember forever, that I can think back on with joy. Walking is the highlight of the day. If I get exercise, great, but that's only a side effect. I won't remember the days I walked more than 10,000 or 12,000 steps, only the days when my walks improved my psyche, gave me treasured memories, wrote entire articles and chapters, the walks that were most joy-filled.

I return to the quote by Henry David Thoreau in Chapter 1, "But the walking of which I speak has nothing in it akin to taking exercise, as it is called, as the sick take medicine at stated hours— as the swinging of dumbbells or chairs; but is itself the enterprise and adventure of the day."

I feel dozens of walks coming on and I live in hope that you do, too.

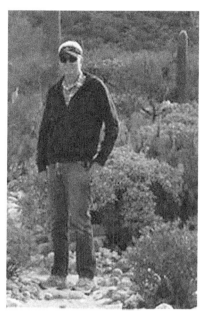

About the author

Robert Cain is an old hand at this writing business and still trying to get good at it. He has authored seven books and writes articles that appear monthly. Two books, plus this one, are available on Amazon, *Get It Rented* and *Evictions: How to Win (or Lose) Them*. All his previous books were about property management, something he wrote, spoke, and conducted trainings about border to border and coast to coast for 30 years along with publishing the *Rental Property Reporter* and *The Northwest Landlord*. Those two publications followed the property management industry and provided information to help property owners and managers manage their rental properties more profitably.

With this book, he went off on a tangent. He has always been an avid walker as is described in various chapters in *The Book of Walking* and has written the book to describe why walking is such a treat, and with the hope that people who read the book will discover that walking for reasons other than exercise are more rewarding.

A 20-year resident of Oro Valley, Arizona, he moved there after living in Portland, Oregon. He lives with his wife, who has tolerated him for more decades than she would have been expected to. He has two grown children and two grown grandchildren, all of whom he is extremely proud.

He'd love to hear from you by email at bob@cainpublications.com.

Made in the USA
Monee, IL
23 December 2022

23420237R00105